MAY   2021

WATER UP
FIRE DOWN

WATER UP FIRE DOWN

An Energy Principle
for Creating Calmness, Clarity,
and a Lifetime of Health

ILCHI LEE

BEST
LIFE
M E D I A

BEST
LIFE
M E D I A

459 N. Gilbert Rd, C-210
Gilbert, AZ 85234
www.BestLifeMedia.com
480-926-2480

Please understand that this book is not intended to treat, cure, or prevent any
disease or illness. The information in this book is intended for educational
purposes only, not as medical advice. Always check with your health professional
before changing your diet, eating, or health program. The author and publisher
disclaim any liability arising directly or indirectly from the use and application of
any of the book's contents.

First paperback edition: November 2020
Library of Congress Control Number: 2020944838
ISBN: 978-1-947502-19-2

Cover and interior design by Kiryl Lysenka

Table of Contents

Own Your Health for Everyone's Sake

I wrote this book in the middle of and in response to the COVID-19 pandemic. This situation has caused great upheaval, pain, and suffering, but we are all in the process of learning an important lesson: we must defend and protect our health—not only for ourselves, but also for our families and our communities.

It was shocking to see the pandemic bring all of humanity to a standstill in a matter of months, even affecting inhabitants of the Amazon rainforest—one of the earth's most remote regions—as well as those living in cities. I felt a need to offer something to the world, something to bring health and healing to people. I wrote this book out of a desire to help people understand ways to protect their health and the health of the planet and to apply in their lives the fundamental principles of energy.

We've seen so many dedicated health care providers who have risked their lives during this pandemic. They are the heroes of our times, courageous people who have shown us the greatness and beauty of the human spirit. Yet, the medical and public health systems could only go so far in protecting us from the virus. Experts could only issue warnings and suggest behaviors, like wearing masks and social distancing, to help "flatten the curve." At the time I am writing this book, medical researchers are racing to find a vaccine and a truly effective treatment. For the most part, we have all been left on our own to take care of ourselves—and each other. The coronavirus woke us up, making us realize that the social systems we've been relying on, medical and political, are more vulnerable than we thought.

It is crucial that we build a medical system that is better able to cope with these situations. However, we can't depend only on health care providers and politicians to prevent disease, allowing us to escape from anxiety to find peace of mind. Each one of us must own our health.

The World Health Organization lists more than 40 types of infectious diseases. The speed at which new contagious diseases arise is gradually increasing, so it's highly likely that we'll face even greater risk in the future. What's more, many scientists are concerned that contagious diseases will spread more as a result of climate change and damage to the natural environment.

Taking care of our own health in our daily lives is the most powerful tool for protecting us from pandemics. People with robust immune systems who caught the coronavirus were able to beat it, while people with underlying disease or weaker immunity were more likely to succumb to the virus.

You probably took your vitamins more diligently than usual during the pandemic and looked for foods said to be good for boosting immunity. But there are no foods or drugs that boost immunity in one shot. The key to good health is maintaining harmony and balance, and that is true for immunity, too. Our immunity is determined by how we manage our bodies and minds on a day-to-day basis, not by expensive new drugs or special foods.

We have within us a wonderful inner physician working to keep us healthy: the immunity and natural healing power built into our bodies and brains. Yet even if our bodies have powerful immune systems, they will naturally weaken if we live in ways that inhibit rather than assist the work they do. Eating and sleeping well and having peace of mind are essentials for good health, as we all know. The principles for enhancing immunity are not much different than the general principles for good health: If you ignore these basics and overwork your body and mind, breaking life's balance and rhythm, your immune system will weaken. Immunology experts unanimously agree that this is true.

The Basis of True Wellness

The World Health Organization designated COVID-19 as a pandemic because of its surprising speed of transmission and high mortality rate. When we look into our daily lives, though, we find many factors that may threaten our health as much as or even more seriously than the coronavirus.

What do the experts consider major factors weakening immunity? They include lack of sleep, lack of exercise, unbalanced eating habits, overwork, stress, alcohol consumption, and smoking. As the world has adopted an industrialized lifestyle and culture, these harmful habits have become a part of many people's lives in most countries. Although such habits severely eat away at our health and immunity, they get less attention than a pandemic because their impact manifests slowly and is not immediately apparent. Diabetes, obesity, hypertension, and heart disease are typical lifestyle diseases. Many of those who have lost their lives from the coronavirus, unfortunately, had such underlying disorders.

Medicine has developed greatly, yet the number of people suffering from such lifestyle diseases is increasing, which confronts us with these questions: Why is it so hard for us to change lifestyle habits that ruin our health, even though we want to be healthy? Why are we negligent about taking care of our bodies in our daily lives when we're well aware of the importance of prevention?

One of the most significant reasons for this, in my opinion, is that we've lost our sense for connecting and communicating with our bodies. We're investing more time and money in our bodies than at any other time in history. Paradoxically, however, we're growing more distant from them. Many people craft their ideal bodies, but they don't actually have a good feel for the state of their health. They aren't paying attention to the signals from their bodies that tell them that their balance is broken. Many even hate their own bodies when they fail to meet the beauty standards set by society.

I believe we should all love and cherish our bodies, regardless of their appearance. They are miraculous, and they deserve our respect. Rather than looking in the mirror to examine them for imperfections, we should learn to feel them, listening for the messages they are giving us. We need to acknowledge the connection between our bodies and minds, and we learn to understand ourselves in the process. This is the basis of true wellness, and it is my reason for writing this book. Our society needs people with healthy minds and bodies, but too often the opposite is true.

What You Can Expect from This Book

I've traveled the world for more than 40 years teaching people how they can create healthy, happy lives and find peace of mind. The people I've met have been diverse in country of origin, age, gender, and social and cultural background, but they've confirmed for me that the secret to maintaining a healthy life doesn't differ much from person to person.

The following three elements reflect universal wisdom for good health, as I think of it.

1. Recognize that you are responsible for your own health.

2. Recover your sense for communicating with your body.

3. Develop and consistently practice life habits for maintaining the harmony and balance of your body and mind.

The purpose of this book is to present you with an energy principle for combining these three elements and to provide you with practical tools and tips that will enable you to practice the principle in your daily life. I want to guide you so the principles of energy do not remain at the level of mere knowledge or information and to enable you to develop routines in your daily life—habits of regularly checking the condition of your body and energy and adjusting their balance immediately. You're unlikely to live your whole life without ever being sick, but I wanted to put into this book the most basic of the basics for preventing serious disease and living with good health and vitality.

The energy principle and methods presented in this book are not complicated or difficult to understand. They are simple and easy enough to be understood and used by anyone. It is not my intention, however, to present a Band-Aid prescription that temporarily eliminates symptoms without looking into the roots of the problem. In the end, your health is determined by whether or not you apply even the simple things I've suggested and how steadily you make them a part of your life.

The contents of this book are based on traditional Asian medicine, which views humanity and nature as one and applies the principles of nature to the human body. The book is also based on Sundo, the Korean mind-body training tradition in which my teachings are rooted, and on Brain Education, a system of personal development I've established. In addition, it is suffused with the 40-year experience of millions of people practicing Body & Brain Yoga, which I created to apply energy principles to everyday life.

If you're trying to recover the good health you've lost, this book offers new perspectives on health and will provide you with health-sustaining routines that will stay with you for the rest of your life. If you're healthy and already have a solid regimen for taking care of your body and mind, the energy principle in this book will make your health routines richer and more complete.

Nature Lets Us Adapt and Grow

Nature has the power to bestow sustainability and stability on all things, enabling the whole to maintain harmony and balance. Cosmic order and balance are maintained even amid dynamic change because this power exists. When balance is broken in our bodies, this is manifested as immunity and natural healing power as nature seeks to recover its original equilibrium. This power will keep us from collapsing even amid countless challenges and trials, ultimately enabling us to adapt and show resilience.

This force is greater than our immune systems. Penetrating and connecting all things in existence, this power is what I'll simply call the "great life force of nature." Our immunity improves, of course, and we can live healthy lives overflowing with vitality when the great life force of nature flows unimpeded in our bodies. As you read this book, I hope you will feel nature's life force moving through your body and that you will continue to cultivate the life you truly want by applying the principles in these pages across the whole of your existence.

Life is a series of challenges and changes. A person with a secure center can accept transitions, learning and growing through them, unafraid. But when we have no center, we collapse, shaken by even small shifts. A solid center in life starts with your health, which you develop yourself. Once you master your body, you can master your mind and own your life.

Ilchi Lee
From Earth Village in New Zealand
Fall 2020

PART 1
Energy
Principle

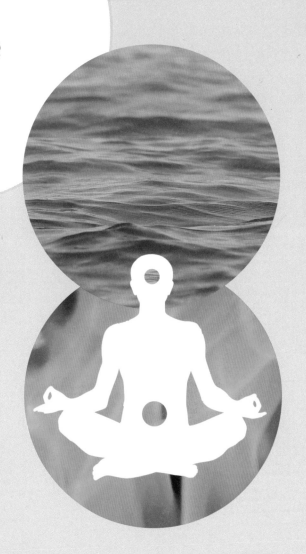

CHAPTER 1

Discover the Golden Principle of Health

I would be foolish to ask, "Do you want to be healthy?" After all, health is the most basic standard for determining your quality of life, and maintaining your health is the greatest gift you can give yourself. Your health is a great blessing for your loved ones and your community, too, since it is the foundation of all the good and beautiful things you do.

You can borrow money and knowledge from others, if necessary, but you can't borrow health. And you can't share your own health with others, no matter how much you love them. Whatever you're seeking to achieve in life right now, you need to base your efforts on *your* health, not anyone else's.

Are you striving for better health? You may be trying different things, such as eating better or exercising more regularly, or maybe you're trying to fix bad habits like smoking or excessive drinking. How's that working for you? Are those efforts bringing you satisfactory results? Do you feel healthy? Or is the gradually deteriorating state of your body causing you to struggle?

Cool Head and Warm Belly

I'd like to introduce a principle that can serve as the cornerstone of your efforts to attain better health, whatever your state of health right now. I call it the "Golden Principle of Health."

First, you must understand that certain principles, or causes, lie behind all natural phenomena. You might also call these principles "natural laws" since they are intrinsic to the way the world works. The reason the sun rises in the east and sets in the west, for example, is that the earth rotates. And the natural law of gravity makes apples fall from their trees. We did not artificially create such natural laws, nor can we change them however we'd like. They have always been there, existing before humans discovered and named them.

Universal principles lie behind our health, too, and failing to live in harmony with them gives rise to illness. With so many people sick these days, illness may seem normal, and it may seem like you have to do an awful lot to keep yourself healthy, but good health is the most natural condition of life. In other words, being healthy is what's normal. So, to regain and retain good health, you need to understand the principles of health and live according to them.

> *"Keep your head cool*
> *and your belly warm."*

This is the Golden Principle of Health that I'm going to tell you about. No matter what physical or mental issues you may have, if you apply this principle in your daily life, you'll be able to make progress toward clearing them up. As a universal law and principle, this applies to everyone, everywhere. You're healthy when you follow this principle, unhealthy when you don't. If you keep ignoring this principle, you may have to pay a hefty price later.

To maintain your health by applying this principle, consider it as important as social distancing, wearing a mask when going out, and frequently washing hands during the coronavirus pandemic. And I want you to make it a daily habit, like eating, brushing your teeth, and washing your face.

Before I describe the principle in detail, let's check your physical condition right now to see how healthy you are in light of this principle. First, use one hand to grasp the arm on the other side of your body. Holding it for two or three seconds, feel the temperature of the arm, and remember that feeling. Now touch your forehead with your hand and then the nape of your neck, sensing the temperature of these two areas. Does your forehead or the back of your neck feel about the same as your arm, or colder? Or does it feel a little or a lot warmer?

Now try feeling your lower abdomen. Try to sense the temperature *inside* your abdomen, not on your belly's surface. Does your gut feel hot or cold inside? Feeling the temperature or sensations in your abdomen may seem difficult for those who have little experience focusing on bodily sensations. If that's you, then it's enough to check the temperature of your hands or feet. Clasping your hands together, try to feel their temperature. Now try sensing the temperature of your feet by touching them with your hands. Do your hands and feet feel warm or cold?

It's great if your forehead and neck feel cool and your belly, hands, and feet feel warm. If that's your condition, you're probably focusing well, with your mind at peace and your head clear. But if your forehead feels hot, or if your lower abdomen, hands, or feet feel cold, then the harmony and the balance of your body may be broken, either temporarily or chronically. In this state—with your neck and shoulders stiff, your body tense, and your eyes and mouth dry—your sensory organs are duller and your breathing is shallower than they should be.

This condition will affect your mental state, as well. In a hurry and flooded with thoughts, you have trouble concentrating. If you try to read a book in this condition, you'll have trouble grasping and retaining its details. So let's stop reading for a moment and change the state of your body. Even if your head is cool and your belly warm, I recommend that you follow the exercise I'm introducing here. Your body will love it.

Sitting (on the floor or in a chair) or standing, make loose fists with your hands. Relax your shoulders and, alternating hands, tap your lower abdomen two inches or so below your navel about 100 times, using the part of your fists where your little fingers are located. Apply enough force that you feel the vibration in your abdominal muscles, providing some degree of stimulation. You should be able to do more than 100 repetitions within a minute. After you finish tapping, close your eyes for about a minute as you comfortably focus on the sensations you feel in your body.

Do you feel a warm heat developing somewhere deep in your belly, spreading to your entire abdomen and lower back? Is your chest more comfortable, your breathing deeper? Does it feel like a kind of pressure or heat in your head is now sinking into your body? Are your eyes moister, and is your mouth filling with saliva? And do you feel better?

The type and intensity of sensations will differ from person to person, but people almost universally feel their bellies growing warmer and saliva filling their mouths. If you're sensitive to physical sensations, you may get tangible feelings of warm vitality filling your body, your vital phenomena being recharged like a depleted cell phone battery plugged into a charger.

It didn't take you even three minutes to do this exercise. You were able to change the condition of your body in a very short time, making your head cooler and your abdomen warmer—in other words, putting your body into a healthier state.

Having a cool head and a warm belly is a good thing; everyone understands this intuitively. Haven't you heard expressions like "keep a cool head" and "build a fire in your belly"? No one welcomes the flushed face that comes from rising anger or the fevered head that comes from having the flu. You probably put a cool towel or ice on your forehead to lower your temperature at such times. You do this because your body tells you what it needs. When you have a bad cold and your whole body is shivering, you don't guzzle cold water or gobble down ice cream. Instead you reach for a bowl of hot chicken soup, or you drink a cup of lemon honey tea—ginger tea in the East—to warm the belly.

An old legend about the eighteenth-century Dutch botanist, chemist, humanist, and physician Herman Boerhaave suggested that this wisdom has been around in the West for quite some time. Dying, he left a sealed book in which he was said to have written the greatest secrets to good health. Many were curious about its contents, but opening the book supposedly revealed text on only a single page. Written in the book was the following: "Keep your head cool, your feet warm, and don't fill your stomach." What's fascinating is that the legendary Chinese doctor Bian Que is said to have left behind those same words about 2,500 years ago. Keep your head cool and your belly warm; these are universal words of wisdom that apply in all times and places.

Why, though, do I go so far as to call this the "golden" rule of health? Our bodies are intricate, complex systems, comprised of many variables. Don't you wonder how I can say that health will automatically follow from observing this common-sense rule?

You have to understand that this principle involves more than "body temperature." It's also about *circulation*. An organism is healthy only if it has good circulation. Only when we have good circulation are nutrients and oxygen supplied to every nook and cranny of our bodies and carbon dioxide and waste products from vital activities fully eliminated.

Many things circulate in our bodies. Blood circulates through our blood vessels, lymph through our lymphatic system, and bio-electrical impulses through our nerves. But there is something crucial circulating through our bodies apart from these things. It's called "energy." The circulation of energy is every bit as important as that of blood and lymph, for it is the foundation that makes all other forms of circulation possible.

"Keep your head cool and your belly warm." This is the Golden Rule of Health because it is the law of *energy circulation*.

Key to Good Health: Energy Circulation

Have you ever received acupuncture treatment? Even if you haven't, you've probably heard about it or seen it in a movie or TV show. Let's say your head hurts so much that it feels like it will explode, and taking medication hasn't helped. You go to see your neighborhood acupuncturist at the recommendation of a friend and explain your symptoms in detail. Strangely, the acupuncturist places needles in your healthy arms and legs without doing anything to your aching head. Even more strange, the throbbing pain in your head vanishes as a result. This kind of thing is possible because Asian medicine looks at our bodies through the lens of *energy.* The acupuncturist views our bodies holistically, their parts interconnected through energy, so he places a needle in your foot to treat a disease of your head and places a needle in your back to deal with a problem in your shoulder.

But what *is* energy? From the calories in the crunchy energy bar you eat as a snack to the head-spinning theories of quantum physics, energy has been understood by scientists in a variety of ways. But the way of describing energy I am using here is much older than that. It's an understanding that is central to Asian medical traditions that are thousands of years old. To put it simply, the energy we deal with in this book is the life force flowing through your body. You could say the concept is similar to that of the bioelectromagnetism created in living cells, tissues, and organs, discovered by Western science, but it is more comprehensive than that. If you're a *Star Wars* fan, you could think of it as something like the Force that surrounds and penetrates us, giving power to the whole universe, the Jedi and the Sith alike.

This energy—commonly called *chi*, *qi*, or *ki*—cannot be seen or touched. That's why some people think it doesn't exist. But just because something is invisible doesn't mean it doesn't exist. Energy exists invisibly, and this unseen thing affects everything visible.

Energy can't be seen with the eyes, but its waves can be felt. (A small minority of people see it, as well.) Organisms have a sense allowing them to feel the subtle flow of energy. How do ants and bats know in advance that an earthquake will occur? Out in the ocean, how do salmon swim such great distances to return to the river where they were born? How do migratory birds get their direction while flying in the wide-open blue sky? Although there are many theories about the fantastic abilities of various animals, the precise mechanisms making them possible remain shrouded in mystery.

Scientists think animals may be using their senses to detect subtle changes in the earth's magnetic field. In fact, although animals may look different on the outside, all are ultimately made of the same stuff—energy. Thus they can detect subtle changes coming from other organisms and objects. This is possible because they feel and respond to energy.

Even without any words being said, we can tell whether a colleague sitting next to us is angry, and we can feel whether someone is overflowing with energy or is sad. That is also energy sensing. We all have a sense for feeling energy, so anyone can develop it further through training. In fact, feeling energy is easier than frying an egg. If you've never experienced feeling energy, please turn to page 184 of this book.

In South Korea, where I was born, going to an acupuncturist to get treatment for shoulder or lower back pain is as common as going to a dentist for a toothache. The idea that pain results from a blockage of energy and that acupuncture can open blockages and improve symptoms is common sense. And it's not just South Korea. The traditional medical systems of Asian countries—which account for close to 60 percent of the world's population—are mostly based on this understanding of energy. Even now, billions of people continue to use such traditional medicine to support their health.

Many people do yoga to lose weight and create a beautiful figure, and they do tai chi or qigong because they've heard doctors say it's good for joint health. But yoga, tai chi, and qigong were original-ly developed by energy masters millennia ago to concentrate and circulate energy in our bodies. Of course, if you have enough energy in your body and it circulates well, you'll also lose weight, and your joints will grow stronger.

In the East, people have long believed that everything in

the world was created by energy. To understand the world, they carefully observed and contemplated how energy acts in nature. They applied the knowledge and wisdom they obtained through observing natural phenomena to the human body because they considered humans to be part of nature. Such experience was accumulated and systemized over thousands of years to become traditional Asian medicine.

> *"It is energy that brings good health*
> *and energy that causes disease."*

This is the most fundamental idea they had in the East concerning the body and health. So to maintain health and heal disease, they first examined and took care of energy. But what should you observe about energy? The primary concern is "circulation."

Just as there are certain patterns even in natural changes that may seem incredibly complex and random, the energy in our bodies moves in certain patterns and directions, not randomly or haphazardly. We're healthy when our energy flows well, without blockages, in its original, natural direction. We develop disease when our energy is blocked or flows in the wrong direction. Symptoms improve and disease is healed when energy blockages are opened up and flow is redirected and corrected. Receiving acupuncture, taking herbal medicine, doing acupressure, or performing certain yoga, tai chi, or qigong movements are all for correcting the flow and circulation of the body's energy.

Water Energy Up, Fire Energy Down

Energy circulation is the key to "keeping your head cool and your belly warm." According to the traditional, natural philosophy of the East, the energy of nature has two opposing essences: *yin* and *yang*. From a yin-yang perspective, what's cool is yin, and what's warm is yang. The properties of energy are further broken down into components commonly known as the Five Elements: wood, fire, earth, metal, and water. Our bodies have pairs of organs governing the operations of each of these Five Elements. The kidneys control water energy, and the heart controls fire energy. Our health is determined by whether or not these two kinds of energy—water and fire—circulate in the correct direction in our bodies, thereby achieving harmony and balance.

One of the most fundamental causes of energy circulation in nature is temperature difference. Energy becomes lighter and rises when heated, and it becomes denser and sinks when cooled. The human body clearly shows this phenomenon in its relationship between circulation and health. When your body is normal, a great deal of blood flows around your abdomen, facilitating the activities of your internal organs, warming your belly, and making its temperature somewhat higher than that of your head. As a result, energy circulation happens automatically, following the natural law by which hot things rise and cold things sink. Energy rising from your warm belly pushes water energy in your kidneys upward, cooling your head; energy coming down from your head, receiving the fire energy of the heart, sinks and heats your lower abdomen, creating a balanced cycle. In Korean, this is called *Suseung Hwagang,* or "Water Up, Fire Down." This system of energy circulation is the foundation of all natural phenomena, not just of the human body.

Translated literally, *Suseung Hwagang* means "water rises, fire sinks." But wait! If it's a law of nature, shouldn't it be the other way around? In a natural state, doesn't water sink and fire rise? Rain

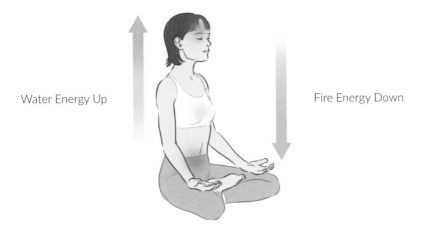

Water Energy Up

Fire Energy Down

WATER UP, FIRE DOWN ENERGY FLOW

falls to the ground, and water flows down from high places to low places. Put a log on a fire, and you'll see that both fire and smoke rise upward. If this question occurs to you, you're not alone. I get this from a lot of people. And you're right. As we learn in natural science classes, hot and light things go up, while cold and heavy things go down. So naturally, fire rises and water sinks. But the opposite movement coexists within a healthy living organism.

Hot, light things rising and heavy, cold things sinking creates the cosmic order and provides stability to everything in existence. Conversely, cold things rising and hot things sinking creates change and provides dynamism.

If there were only stability without creation and change, the hot would continue to stay up and the cold to stay down, making this a dead and unchanging universe. Conversely, if there were only creation and change without stability, the universe would enter an utterly disordered state in which nothing could be predicted.

Creation and change are part of the miracle of life, flowers blossoming amid stability. Countless possibilities being conceived and realized through creation and change within a framework of predictable natural laws is a picture of the great cosmos.

Water Up, Fire Down circulation can be observed in nature as well. The sun's hot rays descend and heat the earth, lakes, and oceans—fire down. Heated water vapor rises to the sky—water up. Trees and other plants use this cycle to survive and grow. Their roots suck up the energy of water from the ground. The leaves receive the energy of fire sent down by the sun. Trees produce leaves and flowers and bear fruit this way through water-fire circulation.

The circulation of water and fire energies is a fundamental life principle of nature. All organisms are healthy when the energies of water and fire achieve good harmony in their bodies, and their life force weakens when this balance is broken. If this principle operates smoothly in your own body, making your head cooler and your belly warmer, you can be naturally healthier.

The vital phenomena of our bodies are maximally activated when we have good water-fire circulation. Picture a healthy baby. Like a tree in spring that's well watered and sprouting bright green leaves, she has a mouth overflowing with saliva, a form of water energy. Her face is soft and smooth, her eyes moist and clear; she's drooling so much it would soak her shirt if she weren't wearing a bib. If you gently place your hand on the belly of a baby who's sleeping soundly and breathing deeply, you'll feel a pleasant warmth coming from her tummy, which rises and falls regularly with every breath.

When the water-fire circulation in our bodies weakens, our vital phenomena weaken as well. Think about the changes that happen as we enter old age. Like trees having lost water energy when the weather grows cold, their branches drying and leaves falling, our faces and skin become dry, rough, and wrinkled; our teeth and hair may fall out; our eyes become dry; our vision blurs; our mouths secrete less saliva; our bodies even lose height. The fire energy of our lower bodies weakens, too, making our bellies cold, our hands and feet often tingling and numb.

When we have Water Up, Fire Down circulation, a state of energy allowing "perfect" health is created. With all systems and organs functioning vigorously, blood and energy circulating well, our bodies overflow with vitality. Since this state facilitates brain activity, the mind is clear, and concentration is focused. We get new, creative ideas. Emotionally, too, we are well balanced and harmonious. In this condition, it is easy to have good relationships with ourselves, other people, and the world.

When your body maintains Water Up, Fire Down circulation, your energy is "open," a state in which energy flows freely, without blockages. In this condition, the best environment is created for your body and brain. This Water Up, Fire Down circulation produces a physiological state in which peak performance is possible in all areas of life—physically, mentally, emotionally, and spiritually. When you feel "I'm in top condition today"—when your head is clear, your mind at peace, your body overflowing with vitality—then the energy in your body is circulating, achieving the perfect balance of water-fire circulation.

"Water Up, Fire Down—keep your head cool and your belly warm." This is the Golden Principle for the health of our bodies. Remember it. Write these words on a sticky note, and post it in an easily visible place. And train so this principle acts in your body, giving you the gift of optimal health.

SUMMARY

- Water Up, Fire Down—Keep your head cool and your belly warm. This is the Golden Principle of Health.

- All organisms are healthy when the energies of water and fire achieve good harmony in their bodies, and their life force weakens when this balance is broken.

- Water Up, Fire Down circulation provides the best energetic and physiological environment for your body and brain.

CHAPTER 2

Balance Your Energy to Manage Your Stress

Has your physical health and mental stability declined because of stress? Maybe you were irritated or angry, anxious or nervous. Your head throbbed, your neck and shoulders ached, or you felt nauseous. You found yourself sighing frequently and feeling weak, you were lethargic and lacked ambition, you were tired and wanted to rest but couldn't sleep. Could you guess what percentage of the day you were in that state, based on the time you were awake—10, 20, 50 percent?

What do you think your energy state was when you were in that condition? Would it have been a state of Water Up, Fire Down circulation, with your head cool and belly warm? Of course not. You could say that your energy was reversed by the same percentage that your physical and mental stability were broken by stress. In other words, your water energy had moved down, making your belly cold, while your fire energy had moved up, making your head hot.

From an energy perspective, stress typically causes a reversed water-fire state, in which the flow of healthy energy is turned upside down. When people get angry or are showing their stress, we say they are "getting heated" or "blowing their top." These sayings are appropriate because when you're angry, the heat energy inside you surges upward, making your face burn and your eyes blaze. Your head becomes like a boiling kettle, its lid rattling because of the bubbling water and the hot steam pouring out. You indeed get heated and blow your top—the expression fits perfectly—when the fire energy surges into your brain.

Let's take a detailed look at what happens in your body and mind when you enter a state of reversed water-fire circulation, with your normal energy flow reversed—fire energy going up and water energy going down.

When Fire Energy Surges to the Head

Let's look at the symptoms that occur as fire energy surges to the head, heating it up.

What people most commonly feel is fatigue of their sensory organs, particularly eyestrain. As fire energy floods the head, your eyes become dry and blurry, and the eyelids grow heavy. Feeling pressure in your eyes, you frown or blink without realizing it. And your saliva secretion decreases, drying up your mouth. Your ears feel clogged and ring, and you may even lose your sense of smell. Your skin becomes rough and dry, making your lips or body scaly.

The next most common symptoms are neck and shoulder tension and headache. The muscles at the back of your head and neck grow stiff and painful, so you have trouble rotating your neck. Your shoulders ache and feel heavy, as if something has been placed on top of them. Your head feels foggy and squeezed, and your temples throb. The back of your neck, your shoulders, and your forehead feel hot to the touch. With heat filling your head, your brain function declines, making you forgetful and hurting your focus—and that results in frequent mistakes. And you end up having trouble sleeping, tossing and turning throughout the night.

Your heartbeat becomes irregular, too, giving you a pounding chest or making you nervous and anxious. You're more sensitive, getting irritated over nothing. Your breathing is shallow and irregular, and your chest feels constricted. Without realizing it, you're often sighing. If your condition is severe, you may develop emotional disorders such as depression. Overall, your emotions are poorly regulated, and you easily become mired in negative feelings.

When your head becomes heated in this way, the pressure in your brain can increase, and its blood vessels can be blocked. This can lead to various nervous system diseases, including mild migraines, facial cramping, eye tremor, tinnitus, and dizziness, and even hypertension and stroke in severe cases.

Picture a land blighted by drought, and it will be easy to understand the symptoms that develop when fire energy accumulates in your brain. Such symptoms are actually the result of a "body drought" that develops when the hot energy of fire remains in the head too long, drying up the cool energy of water in the brain and face. When lack of rain leads to drought in the land, the ground grows dry and barren, the air above it full of choking dust. Then the ecosystem suffers—not only the plants putting down roots in the arid ground but also the animals living off of them. So it is with our bodies. If fire energy stays in the head without sinking, desiccating both body and mind, life starts to fall apart, snapping like a dried branch in winter.

When Water Energy Sinks to the Belly

Now let's look at what happens when water energy sinks down, making the belly cold.

Most of the major internal organs, other than the brain, heart and lungs, are located in the abdomen, including the stomach, liver, large intestine, small intestine, kidneys, and bladder. The belly must be warm for these organs to function well. But if the belly grows cold due to a lack of water-fire energy circulation, the intestines become stiff and sluggish, leading to various diseases of the digestive system. Countless problems can develop such as indigestion, heartburn, gastritis, irritable bowel syndrome, reflux esophagitis, leaky gut, and diarrhea. Bowel function deteriorates, easily leading to constipation.

Additionally, digestive and metabolic functions decline, making it easy to gain weight. People who are obese aren't likely to think that their abdomens are cold since they may often feel hot and sweaty more often than thin people. However, once their senses are enhanced so they can feel their abdominal energy, they sometimes have cold and even icy sensations in their bellies.

A cold belly harms mental health. It is well known that the intestines directly impact one's emotional state. More than 95 percent of serotonin (the "happiness hormone") and 50 percent of dopamine (involved in feelings of pleasure) are produced in the intestines. You have probably experienced becoming more sensitive and irritable when you have a stomachache. Studies have shown that poor intestinal health can lead to anxiety, depression, and autism, as well as Alzheimer's disease.

Seventy percent of the cells conferring immunity in our bodies are in the intestines. When water energy floods the abdomen, making it cold and reducing intestinal function, immunity is weakened, resulting in frequent colds and susceptibility to various diseases such as cancer. A colder abdomen also weakens reproductive functions. Women may have menstrual irregularities and pain, or they may develop uterine tumors, which negatively impacts conception. Sexual function declines in both men and women.

The symptoms that develop with the buildup of water energy in the abdomen might be compared to what happens during an unexpectedly long rainy season. Rain is essential, but there's nothing more inconvenient than a drawn out rainstorm with never-ending downpours. Waterways overflow, swamping the fields where grains once grew and causing wild animals to lose their habitats. A continuing rainy season makes houses humid, bringing unpleasant smells and spreading mold. Similarly, our bodies become heavy and sluggish, and our minds become depressed if we experience too much rainy weather. If you've experienced such a downpour, do you remember wanting the rain to stop and the sun to shine and burn off that damp energy? When our bellies are filled with water energy, cold and soggy, our bodies experience the exact same "energy rainstorm" and want to escape it.

Energy Circulation and Stress

We've listed in detail the phenomena that arise when the flow of energy in our bodies is reversed. Don't these seem really familiar, as if you've already experienced or heard about them a lot? That's right—they're virtually identical to the symptoms we experience when we're under stress. Stress and reversed water-fire circulation have a relationship like that of the proverbial chicken and egg. They are so closely related that it is difficult to determine which comes first—which is the cause and which is the effect. Being under stress reverses your energy flow, and a reversal of energy flow puts you under stress.

As you already know, stress is the greatest threat to a happy, healthy life. According to the American Medical Association, stress is the cause of 80 to 85 percent of all disease. Stress, if unmanaged, places people at greater risk for cancer and heart disease than smoking or high-cholesterol foods, according to a study conducted over 20 years by the University of London.

Various studies have also shown that stress has a major negative impact on the immune system. People experiencing severe stress disorders are 30 to 40 percent more likely to have autoimmune diseases than the general population, according to a study analyzing the medical and health data of 1.28 million people in Sweden. A psychology research team at Ohio State University reported that patients with higher levels of stress had 20 to 30 percent fewer white blood cells—which is the foundation of the immune system—than the general population.

Even without scientific evidence, we understand from our own daily experience that stress reduces immunity. Have you ever experienced an outbreak of cold sores or pimples or suffered from a fatigue-related illness after a long struggle with some stressful project or event?

Not only does stress lower our immunity and damage our health, but it can also turn us into bad-tempered individuals. No matter how good your character, it's hard to remain a good person if you're up to your eyeballs in stress and stuck with reversed water-fire circulation for a long time. Even those who might be called "gods of positivity" have a hard time extracting themselves from the swamp of negative thoughts and emotions when they've been under the influence of reversed water-fire circulation for a lengthy period. Angry without really knowing why, they develop an attitude that says to the world, "Nobody better mess with me!" As if wearing gray-filtered glasses that make everything look gloomy, they feel harassed by everyone around them.

When we are healthy, the water-rising, fire-sinking pattern is an energy balance that appears spontaneously as a result of natural energy circulation. Usually the large volume of blood circulating through the midsection automatically warms the belly to promote the activities of the internal organs. Energy circulation happens all on its own because the abdomen is relatively warmer than the head. When we're healthy, our bodies do what they should to maintain proper water-fire circulation.

But when we're in a stressful situation, blood flow concentrates in our arms and legs, readying us to take action in what's called the "fight or flight response." As this happens, heat builds up in the brain, and the temperature of the abdomen falls. If this continues, reversed water-fire energy flow develops, heating the upper body while cooling the lower region.

In modern times, as the chronic stresses of daily life have increased, maintaining Water Up, Fire Down energy circulation has become more and more of a challenge. Just thinking about how much stress surrounds us will give you an idea of how easy it is to get stuck in a reversed water-fire energy state. Our lifestyles are practically stress-manufacturing machines that flip our energy flow several times a day, giving us hot heads and cold bellies.

You know that stress is the source of all kinds of diseases, but living without stress isn't possible. This isn't true only for school and work life, where we have to deal with competition, evaluation, targets, and deadlines, but also for our relationships with family and lovers, where we are bound to fight over differences of opinion. And many external stressors are simply beyond our control. COVID-19 has been a worldwide stressor no one could avoid, no matter how rich, powerful, or famous he or she might be.

Of course, not all stress is bad. Appropriate tension empowers you to overcome difficulties and accomplish your plans, energizing your life. According to people who study stress, you may actually develop more disease if you excessively *avoid* stress or live in an environment where stress is extremely limited.

Our body's stress response is designed to help us survive external threats. You and I wouldn't be here today if our primitive ancestors felt no stress when charged by a lion, instead continuing to enjoy the taste of the raspberries in front of them. If we weren't stressed at all by approaching deadlines, could we finish our projects on schedule? We have been evolving through a process of adapting to stimulation and change—in other words, while under stress. The process of coming out into the world after being in our mothers' cozy wombs, where everything was provided, was incredibly stressful for our mothers and for us. We were given life through that process. Accepting stress as a part of life and dealing with it proactively is much wiser than unconditionally avoiding it, thinking of it as an enemy.

Strategies for Managing Stress

Two things help us manage stress well. First, developing resistance to stress lets our bodies and minds be less negatively affected by stressful situations. Second, cultivating techniques for quickly releasing stress prevents stress from becoming chronic. In other words, handling stress effectively involves experiencing less stress and quickly resolving whatever stress we can't avoid.

Responses to stressful situations differ depending on the individual, even in the exact same situation. When given an opportunity to make a presentation to an audience of thousands at a national conference, some would feel positive excitement and expectation, while those with a fear of public speaking would experience panic-inducing stress. When busy and stuck in traffic on their way to work, some people lose their composure, honking and cursing at cars that cut in front of them, while others remain calm.

Wouldn't it be great to develop resistance to stress, moving from mental fragility and being overwhelmed by even slightly stressful situations to mental toughness, finding the resilience to adapt and deal flexibly with most of the stress you're likely to face? Water Up, Fire Down energy circulation creates the mental steel that lets you remain unshakable in any circumstance and have the constancy to boldly go your own way and not be swept away by the waves and vicissitudes of life.

Time is the key factor that turns stress into disease. Even if you're under great stress, you'll be okay as long as you recover well, but your mind-body balance collapses even under mild stress if it continues for a long time. For example, the death of a family member, while shocking, is a stress that naturally subsides with time. But the little stresses occurring every day on the job and at home more easily lead to disease if they build up without being resolved. That's why you need to recognize the importance of managing stress and develop a habit of resolving stress in your daily life without letting it build up.

When you went to bed last night, how much of the day's accumulated stress did you take with you? When you start a new week, how much still remains of the stress built up over the previous week? When you're placed in a stressful situation, how long does it take you to adapt to or overcome the feeling of stress? Do you have a habit of resolving stress in a healthy way rather than ignoring it and letting daily stresses pile up until they are an obstacle, both physically and mentally? Or do you use less healthy ways to manage stress, turning to comforts such as overeating or drinking, which take their own toll in the long run?

You can recover from fatigue caused by physical exertion by getting some rest, but recovery from stress caused by mental injuries doesn't proceed quite so smoothly. No matter how much you may want to change your mind about something, it's not always easy. Like a car engine damaged by a driver who pointlessly spins its wheels, you try but fail to change your mind, getting more stressed out in the process. There is a powerful principle you can use at this time:

> *"Energy creates mind,*
> *and mind creates energy."*

This means that energy and mind are an inseparable whole, affecting and being affected by each other. If your efforts to change your mind aren't working out so well, try changing your energy. Restore your water-fire energy balance by causing the fire energy in your head to sink and the water energy in your belly to rise. Your body will recover vitality, and your mind will find more peace if your energy state changes in this way.

A good body and a good mind come from a good energy state. It's also much easier to be a good person if you have the right water-fire energy circulation. Water Up, Fire Down isn't only a principle for protecting your health, but it also lets you manage stress and use it as a driving force for positive change and growth.

The Physiology of Water-Fire Energy Circulation

You may have been in a situation where you were driving and had to stomp on the brake when the car in front of you stopped suddenly. Your heart was probably pounding and your breathing most likely became rapid. Your forehead began sweating, your shoulders became tense, and your hands gripped the steering wheel tightly. After realizing you were safe, you probably calmed yourself, exhaling deeply. Such physical reactions, which we usually take for granted, are all operations of the autonomic nervous system. Breathing, sleeping, digesting food, controlling heart rate, regulating body temperature—all these physiological functions happen without our thinking about them because they are regulated by the autonomic nervous system. This system is the key to maintaining the homeostasis, stability, and balance of our bodies.

The autonomic nervous system begins in the center of the brain and spreads out along the spinal nerves. It is divided into the *sympathetic* and *parasympathetic* nervous systems, with one growing weaker when the other grows stronger, like a seesaw. The sympathetic system excites us and makes us tense, while the parasympathetic system causes us to rest and relax. The sympathetic nervous system deals with crises, and when we are under stress, it takes the initiative, controlling our bodies and brains. Meanwhile, the relaxing, detoxifying, and healing functions handled by the parasympathetic nervous system are lessened or temporarily suspended.

When you're alarmed—like when you slammed on the brakes— your sympathetic nervous system is activated. Then your heart rate, blood pressure, and blood sugar rise, and blood leaves your digestive and other internal organs, concentrating in the large muscles of your arms and legs. The blood flow in your muscles can rise as much as 1200 percent to give your arms and legs the energy they need to get you out of a crisis situation quickly.

Once the stressful situation ends, your parasympathetic nervous system kicks in, stabilizing your body, which has been in crisis mode. One part of the parasympathetic system is the vagus nerve—the longest of the cranial nerves, with the most complex distribution. Beginning in the brain, it passes the throat and esophagus, spreading to the organs of the thoracic and abdominal cavities—the lungs, heart, stomach, liver, small intestine, large intestine, and kidneys. The vagus nerve acts to slow the heart rate and creates enzymes to promote digestion. It ensures that the kidneys create urine and that food is digested vigorously in the small intestine. It also stimulates the tear and salivary glands.

The sympathetic and parasympathetic nervous systems maintain harmony and balance in our bodies, giving and taking, cooperating like incoming and outgoing tides. Stress, though, is continuously increasing in our daily lives, and that frequently breaks the balance between these two systems. In our modern era, the sympathetic system dominates too much of the time. As a result, the body's stress reaction keeps us tense and in crisis mode. And as the duration of parasympathetic-system suppression lengthens, our bodies lose the opportunity to recharge.

Sympathetic activation consumes the body's energy, while parasympathetic activation restores it. When the overworked sympathetic nervous system keeps using energy, it can't properly recharge so that later the body starts breaking down here and there. If this keeps repeating, the body's muscles, nerves, and organs become fatigued, blood circulation declines, immunity drops, and endocrine function is disrupted. All kinds of diseases develop as balance—the very heart of good health—is upended and the body loses its ability to self-regulate.

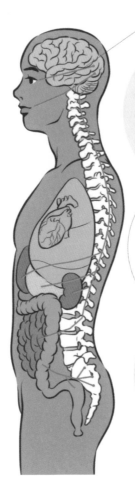

Eyes

As water energy reaches the head, the eyes become moister, stagnant energy and toxins release through tears, vision may seem clearer.

Vagus Nerve

Mouth

Circulation of water energy in the head produces saliva; stagnant energy releases through yawning.

Heart

Heat in the heart is released as fire energy travels down toward the abdomen. Heart rate stabilizes.

Lungs

Breathing becomes deeper and slower, bringing in more oxygen and releasing carbon dioxide.

Abdomen

The abdomen becomes warmer as fire energy accumulates and the digestive tract moves more easily. Blood flows more readily.

Kidneys

The kidneys generate water energy from the fire energy that reaches it.

ENERGETIC AND PHYSIOLOGICAL CHANGES
WITH WATER UP, FIRE DOWN

To return our bodies to a state of balance, we must reduce the burden on our overworked sympathetic system and activate our suppressed parasympathetic system. It's particularly important to activate the vagus nerve, which is connected to our major organs.

Typical responses that occur when we have good water-fire energy circulation—the belly warming, heart and respiratory rates slowing, eyes growing moist, mouth filling with saliva—are physiological phenomena seen when the parasympathetic nervous system, in particular the vagus nerve, is activated. In other words, by creating a state of water-fire energy circulation through our personal efforts, we can restore our autonomic balance. And this natural energy circulation—by activating the parasympathetic nervous system—can bring rest and relaxation to a brain and body tensed and agitated by stress.

SUMMARY

- When water-fire energy flow reverses, with a hot head and a cold belly, the quality of all areas of life drops.

- When hot energy surges into your brain, you experience eyestrain, stiff neck and shoulders, headaches, irregular heartbeat, and a foggy mind.

- When water energy pools in your belly, you develop various digestive and mental health problems, including anxiety and depression.

- Maintaining Water Up, Fire Down energy circulation is an effective strategy for managing your stress.

CHAPTER 3

Connect with Your Body to Prevent Disease

Our bodies have a variety of mechanisms for maintaining harmony and balance. For example, our bodies automatically regulate body temperature, blood pressure, blood sugar, and heart rate, and our immune systems protect us from bacteria and viruses. Our bodies are exquisitely sensitive and intuitive, maintaining their own balance and harmony and signaling us when that balance is broken. These signals may show up as muscle tension or pain, or even as emotions such as nervousness, lethargy, or melancholy. When your body sends you such signals, it's important to listen and take care of it.

However, most of us fail to recognize the signals because we are disconnected from our bodies, living with our attention focused on the outside world instead of on our bodies. With our senses entirely dulled, we can't recognize the signals our bodies are sending. And we ignore the signals we do recognize, telling ourselves that they aren't a big deal or that we are too busy to do anything about them.

Even with our neck and shoulders aching, we're in the habit of sitting in front of a computer all day, putting up with the pain.

For many people, the world inside of the computer captures their attention even more than the world they live in. For hours at a time, they answer emails, binge watch videos, obsess over social media, and play video games. Though their bodies are screaming, "Stand up! Take a walk!" they just keep sitting there with their eyes transfixed on the screen.

Others overindulge on food and drink. Sometimes, they even plan ahead, stocking their medicine cabinets with antacids and hangover remedies. Others recklessly follow fashionable diets without considering their physical condition. Then, they habitually swallow pain relievers when they feel discomfort in their bodies, without looking carefully at what is causing the pain.

To apply the principle of water-fire energy circulation in daily life, you must stop and listen to what your body is saying. Read the signals telling you the condition of your body. Is your head hot or cool? Are your belly, hands, and feet warm or cold? Is your breathing comfortable and deep, or short and shallow? Do you have any tense, knotted muscles? Is your posture straight or bent? It's important to look closely at these things.

You can take action to recover balance only if you realize that your body has lost it. This is a matter of identifying what your body needs and acting upon that information—drinking water when you're thirsty, cutting back on food when you've had too much to eat, supplementing your diet when it lacks nutrients, exercising or stretching when your body feels stiff and sore, getting some sunshine when your body lacks energy and feels cold, and getting a massage or plenty of rest when you have accumulated fatigue. Unless you realize the condition of your body, you won't know what it truly needs, resulting in a gradual worsening imbalance.

If you are indifferent to your condition and are waiting until you can no longer take the pain, you are inviting your condition to become much more serious or even chronic. It is much better to act now on behalf of your health by learning to pay attention to its needs and responding to them today.

A Body with Water-Fire Energy Circulation Rejects What's Unhealthy

Following the Water Up, Fire Down principle might just help you get rid of those bad habits you've been trying to fix for years. Students in the Body & Brain Yoga energy training system I have created are sometimes able to change their habits in a short period of time using this principle.

One of my students, Jane, started smoking when she was in college, so it was a deeply ingrained habit of almost 20 years. On stressful days, she smoked two packs. She tried, unsuccessfully, to quit smoking after she married and had children, if only for the health of her kids. Wondering why she couldn't quit when others seemed to have done so, Jane developed low self-esteem, thinking of herself as a hopelessly weak-willed loser who was beyond saving. But barely a month after she started practicing Body & Brain Yoga, Jane quit smoking—completely. And it's not that she intentionally tried to quit. After just a short time of energy training, she found that smoking now made her nauseous, so she could no longer do it.

There are countless examples of this. A man who once drank alcohol like water, saying he loved the taste, suddenly could not palate the bitter taste. Someone who constantly ate greasy hamburgers could no longer stomach them because of their nauseating, fatty smell. Such individuals all say the same thing: "It's weird, like my body rejects it." But there's nothing weird about it at all. Their bodies' senses have returned to normal. With good water-fire circulation, the body hates and rejects any incoming energy that breaks its harmony and balance.

The Energetic Root of Disease

Western medicine recognizes a condition as disease only if specific symptoms appear—for example, a tumor, bacteria invading the body, extreme pain, or a significant change in vital signs. Traditional Asian medicine, on the other hand, has the concept of *mibyeong*, a state of suboptimal health leading to disease. Mibyeong refers to an unhealthy condition that isn't disease in itself but could lead to sickness if ignored. It refers to cases in which, though there is no clear disorder, uncomfortable symptoms continue. For example, you might feel severe fatigue every time you get up in the morning or get no relief from fatigue even though you've had plenty of rest. Your body might shiver and ache all over, chilly but showing no clear cold symptoms. You might have frequent indigestion or trouble sleeping. If you're a woman, your menstruation schedule or volume might change frequently.

Records of the Grand Historian, the work of Sima Qian, a famed Chinese historian from the early Han Dynasty, contains this mibyeong anecdote. The king of Wei called on renowned physician Bian Que and asked him, "I've heard that you and your brothers are all skilled in the medical arts, but which of you is the best?"

"The eldest brother is the most skilled," said Bian Que. "Followed by the second, and then me, the most inadequate." Wondering at this, the king asked, "Why, then, are you the most famous?"

"My eldest brother treats a patient's disease, eliminating its cause, even before its symptoms appear," Bian Que responded. "My second eldest brother treats a disease early in its onset. So their medical arts are only considered useful for treating minor diseases. I finally recognize and treat diseases only when they are already so critical that people feel pain. This is why I, the least skilled of us three brothers, am rumored to be an excellent physician." In other words, Bian Que's eldest brother treated mibyeong, the condition before actual disease arose, while Bian Que waited until there was a full, chronic disease condition.

A healthy body may momentarily lose and then recover balance, experiencing a reversed energy circulation before returning to the healthy water-fire pattern. When you come home after working all day, for example, your head may be hot, and you may feel tired. This is even more likely on especially stressful days. But after you rest and get plenty of sleep, you return to normal. Your heated head is cooled during the night by water-fire circulation.

When we're healthy, all our vital activities occur naturally. We have good digestion, breathe comfortably, sleep well, and move without pain. It's normal for your body to be light and free of dis-comfort when you get up in the morning. However, if your head is foggy, your breathing uncomfortable, and your body heavy even though you've had enough sleep, and if that lasts for days, then you've developed chronic, reversed water-fire energy circulation.

Busy focusing on work, we typically ignore this unhealthy state; our condition isn't good, but it isn't bad enough to go to the hospital. This leads to a repeating cycle of being tired and sluggish in the morning and having little ambition when the afternoon rolls around. With fatigue continuing to pile up, you finally go to see a doctor, worried because your uncomfortable symptoms have gotten worse instead of better. A doctor examines you, and perhaps you get an ECG, blood tests, X-rays, and all kinds of tests. You feel that your condition is clearly getting worse, but—frustratingly—the doctor says there's nothing physically wrong with you.

If this sort of thing is repeated several times, your body grows accustomed to being stiff and tired, and you get used to being lethargic and having little ambition. You start to believe that this is just how everybody lives. "I've always been this way," you think, and without even realizing it, you end up trapped by your own hypnosis. Being in poor condition becomes your normal daily experience, with your immunity reduced and your body less resilient.

While your doctor won't diagnose this condition as a disease, from the perspective of water-fire circulation, it's a diseased state of energy—one in which a problem has developed in your energy circulation system. The water-fire energy circulation of your body is weakened so that even a little stress reverses its energy flow; it takes a long time for the reversed energy to return to normal.

Sickness doesn't develop in a single day. Virtually no disorder is absent one day, only to appear suddenly the next. It's merely that we've ignored the state of our body, being unaware of the problem or, even if we were aware of it, not knowing what it was. Of course, there are bacterial and viral infections and diseases that have an acute onset, like COVID-19, but these are more noticeable and short-lived. Most serious illnesses progress slowly over a long period of time, and they are bound to be accompanied by warning signals great and small before developing into chronic diseases.

Do you know how long it takes a single cancer cell to grow into a tumor just one centimeter in diameter? It takes about 10 years, according to doctors. By the time one cancer cell grows into a billion cells, it has become a lump about a centimeter in diameter and weighs about one gram. Only when it reaches this size can it be diagnosed through examination or radiographic testing. The 10 years or so that it takes for the cells to grow to the size at which diagnosis is possible can be considered the incubation period for all cancers. Cancer is so scary because it takes a decade to reach one centimeter but then barely a year to double in size because the number of cancer cells grows exponentially. The cancers that shock us because they're discovered unexpectedly do not, in fact, just suddenly appear one day. Instead, many years of imbalance within the body gave rise to the condition.

It's easier for your condition to go back to its original, normal state before a disease has already shown itself. Uncomfortable symptoms appearing in our bodies and minds are physical signals, our bodies telling us that their energy is blocked and asking us to remove those blockages. If we recognize such signals early on and correct the flow of energy, we can stop these conditions from developing into severe diseases. But if energy stagnation continues for a lengthy time, pain and discomfort will increase, leading to severe physical and mental disease.

Vitality and Resilience Should Be the Norm

When we develop physical and mental discomfort, there's always some reason for it. Although it's crucial to get the help of medication or health care professionals to resolve any symptoms that have appeared, it's also important to examine your daily life, the fundamental cause of those symptoms. Look carefully at whether you have any habits or patterns moving you away from balance of body and mind. No one else can do this for you. Someone else can give you advice, but you alone can pay yourself loving attention, being kind and caring to your own body and mind, which will be with you for the rest of your life.

As our life spans increase, personal health and well-being are coming to the forefront as never before. Nobody wants to live a long time in a state of sickness. And long gone is the passive way of thinking of health as merely a state free of disease. The trend these days is to pursue a condition in which your body and brain provide you maximal support, enabling you to do all the activities that give you joy and fulfillment, a state of optimal health balanced in all dimensions of life—physically, emotionally, mentally, and spiritually.

Don't think it's normal to lack resilience because chronic stress has caused a decline in your body's recuperative power. That's definitely not normal. In that condition, your energy becomes heavy and resists change rather than accepting it—stagnating and pooling, failing to flow in a way that will make your life free and powerful.

We have a perfect energy system that lets us display the functions of our brains and bodies at their best. Use the Golden Rule of Health to activate the energy system built into your body, instilling your life with new vitality and resilience. Water Up, Fire Down will create an optimal environment for life, allowing you to joyfully immerse yourself in your work and personal relationships, and to realize the values you hold dear. It will enable you to discover in yourself the power to go your own way, boldly and confidently, without losing faith in yourself no matter what others may say. And it will give you the strength to endure when the world knocks you to the floor and the resilience to bounce back, empowered as never before.

SUMMARY

- To apply the principle of Water Up, Fire Down energy circulation to your daily life, stop and listen to what your body tells you.

- With good water-fire circulation, the body naturally rejects any incoming energy that would break its harmony and balance.

- Use the Water Up, Fire Down energy principle to protect your health when in a state of mibyeong (not yet a disease, but could lead to sickness if ignored).

CHAPTER 4

Run Three Engines for Water-Fire Energy Circulation

B efore we start learning specific methods for recovering Water Up, Fire Down circulation, let's take a closer look at the energy system where this circulation occurs.

Have you ever gone to an acupuncture clinic and seen a model of the human body with lines and points all over it? The lines indicate the paths along which energy flows, and the points show where it enters and leaves the body. Those energy pathways are called "meridians." Like interconnected subway lines moving passengers from place to place in a city, meridians are connected vertically and horizontally, carrying energy to every corner of our bodies.

Along the meridians are points where energy is concentrated and where it enters and leaves the body. These are called "acupuncture points" or "energy points." You could think of energy points as switches or valves for regulating the flow of energy passing through the meridians. You can control the flow of energy along the meridians by placing needles in these points, by using moxibustion or acupressure, or by adopting specific postures or movements. Our bodies have 12 major meridians associated with each of the organs, as well as eight extraordinary meridians, with two of these eight meridians flowing along a central line at the front and back of the body. We also have 365 energy points.

But you may be wondering, "Why can't I see these meridians and energy points?" No sign of them can be found anywhere in the body, even with dissection. So how were they discovered, and how were the theories relating to them developed? How were standardized treatments created indicating which meridians and energy points to stimulate when certain diseases are present?

The answer is that they were developed slowly over many millennia through people's direct experience with energy. For thousands of years, many cultures, especially Asian cultures, have created theories about energy and have developed practices for cultivating and feeling energy. Tai chi, qigong, and yoga are examples of these practices that you may recognize, but there are many more, as well. Typical Asian medicine treatments, including acupuncture and acupressure, developed through many years of direct experience. Theories and practices concerning the body's energy system were established as the evidence of thousands of years was added to information developed by ancient sages, yogis, and qigong practitioners. This was based on what they had seen with their own eyes, felt with their bodies, or understood intuitively through deep meditation and ascetic practices.

Two of the meridians in our bodies are directly associated with water-fire energy circulation. In Asian medicine, these are called the Governing Vessel and Conception Vessel meridians. The Governing Vessel Meridian represents the yang, masculine, and fire aspects of the body, while the Conception Vessel Meridian corresponds to the yin, feminine, and water aspects. But to emphasize the body's ideal flow of energy, I will call the Governing Vessel Meridian the "Water

Way" and the Conception Vessel Meridian the "Fire Way," because the Governing Vessel Meridian is where water energy goes up to the head, and the Conception Vessel Meridian is where fire energy goes down to the abdomen. These two meridians flow along the back and front of the body like two sides of the same coin.

First, the Water Way (Governing Vessel) starts at your perineum—the area between the genitals and the anus—and rises past your tailbone and along your spine to the back of your neck. From there, it rises along the back of your head to your crown, and then goes down past your forehead and nose until it stops at your upper lip. The Fire Way (Conception Vessel) starts in the indented place below your lower lip, passes your jaw, neck, chest, and belly, and continues down to your perineum.

The Water Way is associated with your brain, spinal column, and kidneys, and the Fire Way is associated with the major organs at the front of your body—your lungs and heart, the digestive organs in your abdomen, and the reproductive organs at the bottom of your trunk. Thus, the Fire and Water ways are closely associated with the organs essential for maintaining life.

The Three Energy Centers in Your Body

The cool energy of water rises to the head along the Water Way, and the warm energy of fire sinks along the Fire Way. Three places in our bodies act like engines that cause the energy to move in this way. One is in the lower abdomen, another in the chest, and the last in the head. In Sundo, the Korean tradition of mind-body training in which my teachings are rooted, these engines are called *dahnjons*. The concept is similar to the chakras spoken of in the yogic traditions of India. Dahnjon means "field of energy." Think of the dahnjon as a powerful center of energy. Based on their locations, these energy centers are called the lower dahnjon, in the belly; the middle dahnjon, in the chest; and the upper dahnjon, in the brain.

Let's take a look at the characteristics and roles of these three dahnjon positions.

First, place your fingers on a point about two inches below your navel. Try to be aware of the center of your abdomen, inward from that spot. Imagine a furnace there, red flames rising, giving off warm heat and light, and warming your entire lower abdomen. This is the feeling of the lower dahnjon. In Chapter 1, I invited you to tap your lower abdomen with your fists. That was to stimulate lower dahnjon energy. Commonly called the "core" or "power zone" in fitness training, this spot is the human body's physical center of gravity and, energy-wise, home to the body's most primal life force. It has a deep association with the functions of the digestive organs in the abdomen, the kidneys, the urinary organs, and the genitals.

The hot energy of the lower dahnjon, which is associated with the color red, governs our physical health. If this energy is healthy, the lower abdomen is warm, digestion is good, and vitality surges. Blood and energy circulate well throughout the body, warming even the hands and feet, though they are distant from the center. But those whose lower dahnjon energy is weak will have cold bellies, will lack physical vitality, will have weak digestive or repro-ductive systems, and will experience frequent diarrhea. In addition to lacking warm energy in their bellies, their hands and feet are cold because energy doesn't circulate well enough to reach that far. And if the lower dahnjon isn't fully charged, energy circulation and vitality throughout the body will be a problem.

Now, use your fingers to press the spot in the middle of your

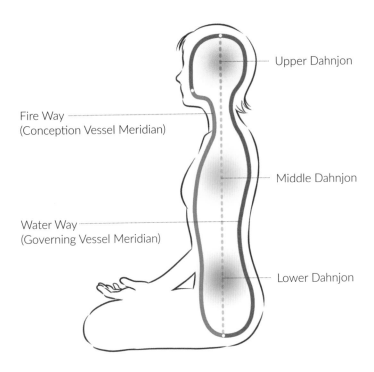

Upper Dahnjon

Fire Way
(Conception Vessel Meridian)

Middle Dahnjon

Water Way
(Governing Vessel Meridian)

Lower Dahnjon

THE ENERGY SYSTEM OF WATER UP, FIRE DOWN CIRCULATION

chest, a slight indentation at the center of your sternum. Inward from there, try to be aware of the center of your chest, the middle dahnjon. Imagine a beautiful, golden rose blossoming there and filling your heart. Golden in color, the energy here is characterized by a comfortable, moderate temperature, neither too hot nor too cold. The energy of the middle dahnjon governs emotional activity. When your middle dahnjon is fully activated, you overflow with confidence and vitality, and you can harmoniously regulate and use your emotions. When the energy of the middle dahnjon is weak, however, you experience volatile emotions and easily find yourself buried in negative sentiments. Your chest becomes tense, you feel stifled or experience a sense of pressure, and your breathing becomes short and rapid. Organs associated with the middle dahnjon are the heart and lungs, along with the digestive organs above the navel—stomach, liver, pancreas, and gallbladder.

Now, touch your finger to the point on your brow between your eyebrows—the place where you see a jewel in the forehead of the Buddha, commonly called the "third eye." Try to be aware of the center of your brain, your upper dahnjon. Imagine a bright star there, giving off a brilliant blue light, brightly illuminating the inside of your head. The energy of the upper dahnjon, blue and cool, governs our mental and spiritual activity. When the upper dahnjon is activated, your consciousness becomes clear and bright, and you develop wisdom, intuition, and insight. But when the energy of your upper dahnjon is weak, then your head is unclear, and you have trouble concentrating or coming up with creative ideas.

Warm Belly, Open Heart, and Cool Head

How do these three dahnjons act as engines in water-fire energy circulation? The foundation of the three is the lower dahnjon, which serves as a center of gravity in our body's energy system, like the base of a pyramid. Just as a pyramid could easily collapse if its base isn't firm, the middle and upper dahnjons could be unhealthy if the lower dahnjon is weak.

When the lower dahnjon is activated, creating a hot energy center in the belly, this energy affects the kidneys in the lower back. According to the Asian theory of the Five Elements, the kidneys are where water energy is created in the body. The hot energy of the lower dahnjon pushes the water energy in the kidneys upward so it rises along the Water Way toward the head, producing circulation—water up.

Rising to the head, the water energy cools and clarifies the upper dahnjon in the brain. Activated by clear water energy, the upper dahnjon refreshes the entire brain. This water energy sinks, moistening the eyes, bringing luster to the face, and causing saliva to pool in the mouth. If excessive mental energy has caused fire energy to build up in the brain, it will be pushed downward toward the trunk.

The heart produces fire energy, and a lot of fire energy is generated and pools in our brains. Having risen from the kidneys, water energy pushes fire energy down from the head and heart, sinking along the Fire Way to the lower dahnjon in the belly—fire down. If water energy fails to push fire energy out of the head and heart, not only does the fire energy stagnate in the head and chest, but in severe cases, the fire energy in the heart reverses direction and rises to the head.

Fire energy coming down from the head and chest and accumulating in the lower dahnjon is delivered to various organs in the abdomen and pushes the water energy of the kidneys up along the Water Way—water up. This is the Water Up, Fire Down energy cycle created by the Fire Way, Water Way, and the lower, middle, and upper dahnjons all working together.

In Sundo, this process of activating the three energy centers is called *Jungchoong*, *Kijang*, and *Shinmyung*. Jungchoong occurs when fire energy has filled the belly. It indicates a physically healthy and energetic state of being. Kijang happens when the energy in the chest has fully matured. Then the heart is completely open and the emotions are balanced. Shinmyung refers to the fully developed energy state of the upper dahnjon in the head. When someone is in a state of Shinmyung, their mental energy is positive and bright. So, when your three energy centers are activated and you have good water-fire circulation, you develop a warm belly, open heart, and cool head. But if your three energy centers are *not* activated and you don't have good water-fire circulation, you end up with a cold belly, closed heart, and hot head.

As we have seen, in terms of energy, Water Up, Fire Down is the most basic foundation of good health and long life, and it is the foundation of effective spiritual practice, as well. In essence, the entirety of our being is influenced by this process of Water Up, Fire Down: the lower dahnjon regulates primal life force and physical health; the middle dahnjon regulates emotions, causing them to mature; and the upper dahnjon handles all mental activities, including clarity and wisdom for life. Thus, consistent development of these three energy centers makes body, mind, and spirit healthier, and that inevitably results in a higher quality of life, as well.

For someone without direct experience of energy, this description of the energy system in our bodies may feel abstract and complicated, making it difficult to grasp. When you sense energy in your body, though, what you feel is as concrete as the taste in your mouth when you eat delicious food, the feeling of food going down your throat, or the happiness that you feel with your whole body. Developing this sense is just like developing any other ability. If you exercise hard, training your abs, you can develop a six-pack. In the same way, if you understand the principles of energy and consistently cultivate your sense for it, you'll be able to feel and strengthen energy centers you were never aware of before.

If you feel energy and continue to develop your sense for it, you'll be able to understand your energy system and the principle of Water Up, Fire Down more deeply, and you'll be able to make better use of the training methods introduced in this book. I believe that everyone should learn how to sense and apply energy for the health of body and mind, just as they might learn how to handle a ball, swim, or do calisthenics in a school gym class.

Even if you can't detect the subtle feeling of energy, the principle of Water Up, Fire Down circulation will help you improve your health and increase your quality of life. The heart of water-fire energy circulation is this: keep your head cool and your belly warm. By checking these right in your body, you can determine whether you have good or reversed water-fire circulation. Your body is like an indicator you always carry with you that can measure the state of your health right away at any time. And if you regularly do the exercises and training for promoting good water-fire circulation presented in this book, you'll start to recover energy balance— breaking through blockages, supplementing energy where you know it's lacking, and reducing it where you have too much. You will be amazed at how efficient a health tool you have—your body— if you start to apply Water Up, Fire Down in your life.

Adding water and heat to raw rice yields something you can eat, but you have to control the amount of water and the intensity of the flame if you want the rice to taste good. Similarly, you'll be able to recover and maintain Water Up, Fire Down circulation in your daily life much more efficiently if you develop a sense for feeling and controlling energy.

SUMMARY

- Water energy travels up through the Water Way (Governing Vessel Meridian) on the centerline along the back of your body.

- Fire energy flows down through the Fire Way (Conception Vessel Meridian) on the centerline along the front of your body.

- Three energy centers in the brain, chest, and lower abdomen work with the two energy channels in the back and front of the body to create Water Up, Fire Down energy circulation.

- When your energy channels and energy centers are fully activated and open, you have a warm belly, open heart, and cool head.

CHAPTER 5

Three Reasons for Reversed Energy Circulation

O ur lifestyles today continually create three situations that block Water Up, Fire Down circulation. First, overheated by our digital lifestyle and information overload, our brains lack time to cool. Second, accumulation of emotional stress in the chest blocks the Fire Way, fire energy's path down out of the brain. Third, unhealthy eating habits and chronic lack of exercise weaken our cores.

Let's take a detailed look at the three trolls that cause reversed energy circulation.

Overworking the Brain Causes It to Overheat

Most of us live lives that are perfect for heating our brains. We think all day, with unmoving bodies and eyes fixed on cell phones, computers, or TV screens. And it isn't only those who sit at desks all day because of their jobs. Most people keep their cell phones close throughout the day. We work, communicate, shop, and now play using our cell phones.

According to a 2016 study by research firm dscout, we touch our cell phone screens an average of 2,617 times during a single day. But that's just the average user. The study found that extreme cell phone users—the top 10 percent—touch their phones more than 5,400 times daily. These figures are four years old, so that number has probably increased quite a bit. The brain can't help but work to process information ceaselessly when we cling to our cell phones and computers except when we're sleeping.

A computer gets "laggy" if you use it for a long time without giving it a break. Overheating slows its response time, reducing efficiency and even causing malfunction in the worst cases. This applies to our brains, too. If you do a lot of mental labor and are under stress, your brain consumes a great deal of energy. So of course, it overheats, resulting in reversed water-fire energy circulation. Your eyes dry out, your head heats up, and your neck and shoulders get stiff and achy. Your concentration drops, too, keeping you from working efficiently.

What do you do when your computer overheats and gets laggy? The best thing is to turn it off and let it cool down. If you always open many apps or activate a bunch of files at once, your computer will become even more finicky, resulting in more problems.

In the same way, it's best to let your brain cool down when it's overheated. But these days we rarely let our brains be, even when they need rest. When we want a break because we're stressed or our heads are a tangle of thoughts, we're likely to say something like this: "I'll just take a minute to let my head cool down."

How do people cool down their heads? A common response is to drink a caffeinated beverage such as coffee or an energy drink. Though these have a temporary awakening effect, they actually stress the brain if used regularly, so more stress accumulates. And typically people reach for their cell phones as they drink their beverage. They scan Facebook or Instagram, watch funny videos on YouTube, check out the latest dance trend on TikTok, or play games. People think they are "taking a break," but their brains are continuing to work at a rapid pace since they are being exposed to a constant stream of information. So, instead of resting and cooling off, the brain consumes more energy, heating up.

What about when people come home from work? Though they say they're tired, people often stay up late playing games, watching TV, or enjoying some other form of entertainment. Even though their brain has already had a long, hard day, they give it more work and cause it to overheat. Our lifestyles steal recuperation time from our brains, time they need for cooling off and recovering from fatigue. If this continues—your brain hot and worn out by fatigue— you won't feel rested even when you do take a break. You'll feel exhausted even when you're not doing anything at all.

Think, too, about the electromagnetic waves coming from computers, cell phones, and portable gaming devices. These "wave-lengths of fire" ceaselessly enter your eyes, so fire energy can't help but flood your brain. Your brain, like a depleted battery, loses its stress resistance, getting hot in no time from even small amounts of stress. At this point, reversed water-fire energy flow has become your default mode.

When excessive heat rushes to our brains, our bodies signal that they want to rest. Our eyes feel tired, our heads heavy, our shoulders stiff, and our minds bored. We're tired and can't concentrate on work even though we've had plenty of sleep. At such times, you need to give your brain a rest by making the fire energy go down. It's easy to end up burning out if you keep running your overheated brain, not letting it cool and ignoring the signals it gives you because your senses have dulled.

Burnout is the severe fatigue and mental exhaustion of a brain that has been completely depleted of emotional energy because of excessive stress. Just as exercising too much causes painful muscles and joints, using your brain too much without recharging it adds to your fatigue and eventually makes you groggy.

Frequent anger, depression, or anxiety are symptoms of a brain that is overheating. These symptoms are warning signals, and if you ignore them and fail to get rest, your burnout will deepen, and you could slide into a prolonged state of apathy and lethargy, a feeling that life has no purpose or meaning.

When you're tired after you've used your body a lot, that fatigue is readily relieved by resting and getting good sleep. But the mental fatigue that comes from overusing your head isn't easily alleviated by resting your body. What should you do, then, to really reduce your brain fatigue? The answer is to cut off the stimulation of information coming from the outside and the thoughts constantly created on the inside, which are the two factors most responsible for causing the brain to heat up.

When your stomach hurts from eating too much food, first you need to stop eating. Taking medication for indigestion may come next. Similarly, the best thing you can do for a brain fatigued and overheated by information overload is to stop all mental activities.

Brain scientists have discovered a specific area of our brains that is actually activated when we rest them, not thinking at all. This is called the default mode network (DMN). Like a computer returning to its default settings when reset, this area of our brains is activated when we rest from mental activities.

The default mode network is vigorously active when you're sleeping or daydreaming, staring off into space—in other words, when there's no external stimulation. When you rest without thinking, your default mode network resets your brain and makes you able to work more efficiently and creatively. When we rest from routine mental activities, our brains reorganize themselves, creating environments that are once again conducive to new activity.

Your brain can better exhibit creativity only when you rest and recharge it. In your own experience, do good ideas and inspiration come from racking your brain and worrying all night? Not likely. Heated all night, our brains yield only thinning hair, rough skin, and dark circles around bloodshot eyes. Instead, good ideas come after we've had enough sleep, maybe while taking a morning shower or going for a walk in the warm sunshine. Didn't Archimedes have an "aha moment" while bathing, and Newton while resting in the shade of an apple tree?

The energy of the upper dahnjon shines more brightly when you have good water-fire energy circulation, which cools your brain. Your upper dahnjon energy lights up, producing clarity, inspiration, and wisdom that lets you see your situation accurately and make good judgments—like a light coming on in a dark room and making objects visible. The upper dahnjon dims, though, when the brain is heated. Then the light of the brain is weakened, hindering discernment—just as it's difficult to distinguish objects in a dark room.

Do you give your brain plenty of rest? Or is a state of reversed water-fire energy becoming your brain's default mode, overheating it? The brain is the commander of the body. If the fatigue of your overheated brain isn't relieved, it will both hurt your health and diminish the quality of your work, personal relationships, and performance across all areas of your life.

Fire Way Blockage Causes a Constant Stifling Feeling in the Chest

The second reason for problems with water-fire energy circulation is blockage of the Fire Way, the path along which fire energy descends. When the Fire Way is blocked, fire energy stagnates in the chest, unable to sink into the belly. With fire energy remaining there, your chest can't help but feel stifled. If you use your head too much or are under stress, that fire energy goes up to your head instead of down, resulting in reversed water-fire circulation.

Here's a method you can use to check the condition of your Fire Way. Start by pressing your forehead with your thumb. Push hard into your forehead, as if you're pushing a tack into a wall. Then use your thumb to make a small circle two or three times, massaging the spot you pressed. Remember how much pressure you are feeling.

Now use the same method to press your chest with your thumb. Start at the bottom of the dent in your neck and go all the way down to the bottom of your sternum, the place where your chest ends. Compare what you feel with what you felt when you pressed your forehead. Pressing your forehead, you probably just had a sense of pressure. When you press your Fire Way, though, there will be places where you feel some pain as well as pressure. Some places will definitely hurt more than your forehead did. Those are spots where your Fire Way is blocked. People with severe blockages may feel enough pain to let out an unintentional yelp, "Ow!"

Don't be surprised that it hurts when you press your Fire Way. Most adults, in fact, have a blocked Fire Way because *everyone* experiences emotional stress, without exception.

Have you ever felt constricted, like something was rising out of your chest, when you were anxious or angry and keeping it to yourself? Then, after you opened up to a friend about your concerns or vented your anger, you felt relieved, as if a lump in your chest had dissolved away. That was because the emotional energy that had been in your chest was released to some extent.

As we live our lives, we experience many things that make us feel angry or hurt, but we can't complain to someone every time that happens. People who do a nice job of managing the energy in their Fire Way are good at identifying and resolving their emotional state when such things occur, not letting troubling feelings build up. Many, however, are not only insensitive to their own emotions, but they let them pile up without expressing their feelings or resolving issues, even when unfair or infuriating things happen to them.

When negative, troubling emotions—anger, worry, fear, sadness, shame, and guilt—accumulate without being resolved, they cause blockages in your chest. With the very center of your Fire Way blocked, naturally the fire energy can't make it down into your belly. Typical symptoms that show up then are feelings of constriction in the chest and difficulty breathing. Your breathing becomes shallow and labored, seemingly blocked in your chest. Your heart may race, or you may sigh constantly without even realizing it. When you are unable to inhale deeply, energy and oxygen don't circulate to every part of your body, reducing your vitality. In that state, you can't control yourself and end up saying a lot more pointless things than usual, or you are easily fatigued even by trivial concerns. With your Fire Way blocked, you also have trouble really opening up your chest. You're habitually bent over, so it's easy to end up with stiff shoulders and a bent back.

According to scholars who study emotion, our various feelings developed because there were reasons for them in the course of our evolution. For example, fear is a survival reaction to protect us in dangerous circumstances. If your house were on fire, without feeling fear you might not think about escaping. Emotions operate faster than reason since they are directly connected with our survival. When we're faced with some situation, our emotions arise reflexively before we even realize what we're up against. Intentionally holding in and suppressing emotions—which are natural, physiological reactions—is definitely not healthy.

Our body's stress reaction was created to protect us from danger. But if it continues too long, our emotions can ruin our health and lower our quality of life—just like the very risks those emotions were designed to protect us from. Negative emotions, especially anger and fear, mostly appear when the sympathetic nervous system is activated in stressful situations. Overly frequent, long-term exposure to such emotions produces excessive energy consumption. It also brings excessive tension to personal relationships. That's why training to appropriately regulate and control emotions is essential.

Of our many emotions, anger is the most destructive because its energy blocks the chest. When anger boils up in the body, respiration and heart rates increase, and blood pressure rises. Breathing becomes rapid and labored, the heart starts racing, the face turns red, and in severe cases, the hands and feet and even the entire body may tremble.

You probably know the power of the physiological responses initiated by the emotional energy of anger. You can feel this not only when you're mad, but also when the person next to you is angry. The fire energy emitted by the body of someone who's angry is transmitted to you, making your heart beat irregularly, your face flush, your body tense and tremble.

"Argh! The more I think about it, the angrier I get," you may tend to say. But when you're all hot and bothered, constantly thinking about it is definitely not a good strategy for resolving the issue that's making you so mad. Let's say you got mad because a work colleague said something insulting about you. The more you think about it, the angrier you get. Your anger is amplified as other episodes come to mind—not only what happened this time, but what happened months ago, years ago. The more you concentrate on those feelings, the more they lead to negative thoughts, which create more negative feelings, continuing in a vicious cycle. Actually, no matter how intense an emotion, its potency is bound to decrease in a matter of minutes—but if you keep focusing on it, the once-weakening flame of that feeling will start blazing brightly again. It's as if you're continuing to pour fuel on the fire of negative emotions while insisting that you want to get away from them.

Emotions are powerful energies that directly impact our bodies and minds. If these potent, emotional energies build up in your heart without being released, they will block your Fire Way, damaging your mental wellness. When you're troubled and mired in negative emotions, if you clutch those feelings, intent on battling with them, you'll lose every time. It's far more efficient to release that emotional energy by opening up your blocked Fire Way.

The Core and the Lower Body Are Weak

The third reason for broken water-fire energy flow is that the lower dahnjon in the belly may become weak. In water-fire energy circulation, the lower dahnjon acts like an anchor holding the fire energy in the abdomen and, like a furnace, making the belly nice and hot. Just as a boat drifts if it's not adequately anchored, fire energy that should stay in the belly rises if the lower dahnjon is weak. And if the dahnjon cools, like a furnace that's not working properly, good water-fire circulation is prevented.

Many things can cause the lower dahnjon to be weak and cold, but the most significant are poor eating habits and lack of exercise. We keep repeating many habits even while knowing they're bad for our health. Fast food can cause our bodies to accumulate unhealthy fat. Processed flour and sugar, high in calories and low in nutritional value, make us gain weight. We don't eat enough vegetables, we eat too much salty food, we eat too quickly, and too often we overeat or gorge ourselves—and all our organs, not just our digestive organs, end up bearing the burden. In addition, our bellies are chilled by our habit of enjoying cold food even in winter—especially cold water or drinks with ice added. Strongly diuretic beverages such as caffeinated coffee and alcohol add cold energy to the body, even while they make us feel momentarily warm.

Virtually no one who lives a sedentary lifestyle—sitting in a chair all day staring at a computer screen, hardly moving their body—has a lower dahnjon that's full of energy. Such lifestyle habits cause your posture to stoop, your blood to pool in your intestines, and your guts to stiffen. In particular, when the fat in your abdomen leads to abdominal obesity, your blood circulation becomes even worse, making your belly colder. Then the functioning of the kidneys, bladder, and other organs decreases, hindering the elimination of waste from your body.

A third of the blood in the body collects in the abdomen. Developing the lower dahnjon is almost like attaching an artificial heart to the belly. When the lower abdomen is warm, blood circulation in the intestines improves, resulting in good flow even to the body's extremities. Fresh blood is supplied to the brain, making the head clearer and improving focus.

In your energy system, the lower dahnjon is the most important foundation. If you're having problems with water-fire circulation, first strengthen your lower dahnjon. When energy is activated in your lower dahnjon—making it hot like a blazing fire and charged with energy—your head automatically cools.

It's important to strengthen the core muscles supporting our bodies. When "core muscles" are mentioned, you may think only of the abdominal muscles, but they also include the muscles of the upper and lower back, buttocks, and pelvis. It's good to strengthen the thigh muscles as well. Your posture is balanced and your internal organs protected only if your core muscles are solid. But when a lack of exercise leads to a protruding belly, stooped posture, and increased body fat, muscles also weaken, as does the intra-abdominal pressure of the belly. Waste products build up, inflammation develops, and the circulation that returns blood to the heart weakens. If your abdominal muscles are in poor condition, lowering the pressure in your abdominal cavity and your core stability, the heat in your head has trouble going down. But when your core muscles are developed, your breathing sinks into your abdomen and further activates the energy in your lower dahnjon.

The way to fix the symptoms that develop as a result of reversed energy flow is to restore Water Up, Fire Down circulation, making it smooth. In other words, all you have to do is correct the things that are inhibiting good water-fire energy circulation. Reduce your thinking to cool your overheated brain, release the emotional energy in your chest to open your blocked Fire Way, and strengthen and warm your belly.

SUMMARY

- Three main factors that create a reversed water-fire energy flow are an overworked brain, a blocked chest, and a weak core.

- To cool down an overheated brain, stop all mental activities, including consuming outside information and entertaining your own thoughts.

- To release the built-up emotional energy in your chest, open up your blocked Fire Way.

- To strengthen the abdomen, work your core and lower body deliberately.

CHAPTER 6

Four Tools for Recovering Energy Balance

I s there anything we can do to correct reversed water-fire circulation in our bodies? Can we do something to maintain a cool head and a warm belly? Fortunately, there are four simple tools that anyone can use to recover Water Up, Fire Down circulation: breathing, meditation, exercise, and awareness. Using these, you can recharge your energy and stimulate your energy circulation.

Control Your Breathing

Breathing is the most powerful yet most basic tool of water-fire energy circulation since breathing is vital for carrying energy in and out of our bodies. We bring fresh energy into our bodies with inhalation and send stagnant energy out with exhalation.

Energy can't be seen with the eyes or touched with the hands, nor can breath itself. But when we inhale, we can *feel* the flow of air coming in through our noses, moving along our airways, entering our lungs, and expanding our diaphragms. And we can *control* our breathing as well as feel it.

It's essential to be able to feel and control our breathing. Why? Through respiration we can control many other things as well.

Suppose you're late for an important meeting. Maybe you're on your way to an interview at a company where you really want to get a job, but a collision leaves you stuck in traffic. You only have 20 minutes left before your appointment, and heavy traffic shows no sign of letting up; it looks like you're going to be late. As you grow anxious, the flow of energy in your body starts to reverse, producing a stress response. Your breathing quickens, your heart pounds, your blood pressure rises, and digestion slows down. This response happens automatically through your autonomic nervous system. You can't intentionally slow your heart, lower your blood pressure, or create more digestive fluid as you might like. But there is one thing you *can* control: your breathing. You can slow your rate of respiration, and you can use it to calm your other stress responses.

What would happen if you exhaled slowly for three or four breaths? Your heart rate would slow, and your blood pressure would come down. You can affect your body's other vital signs, too, by controlling your breathing this way.

Through breathing, we can control more than our body's phys-iological functions. We can control our thoughts and emotions. In a situation like the one I've just described, anyone would grow anxious, with all kinds of negative thoughts arising. You might think to yourself, "That will blow today's interview" or "Why does this always happen to me?" But if you breathe slowly and deeply, your tangled thoughts will subside, and your pounding heart will settle down. You might be able to calmly call your interviewer to explain what has happened and defer your interview.

We move and control energy through our breathing. That's why respiration is the most important tool for managing water-fire energy circulation. But to develop water-fire circulation using this tool, it's important to understand *quality of breathing*.

We always seem to be breathing the same way, but in fact, that's not really the case. Our respiration changes according to our thoughts and feelings, and also according to our age and health. We huff and puff when we're angry, and we sigh slowly when we're sad. We naturally breathe deeply into our lower belly when we're young, but much more shallowly as we get older. If you watch a baby or toddler lying asleep on their backs, you will see their bellies expanding and contracting like a balloon. As we grow older, our breathing moves to our chests, moving only our upper torsos. Finally, when people are close to death due to advanced old age or sickness, their breath rattles in their throats. The less deeply into our bodies we breathe, the more its quality is reduced.

Good respiration for water-fire energy circulation involves inhaling and exhaling deeply and slowly into the lower abdomen. This is called abdominal breathing. Abdominal breathing first expands the entire chest cavity, the diaphragm moving up and down to bring as much oxygen as possible into the lungs and efficiently discharge carbon dioxide. The movement of the diaphragm up and down then becomes more vigorous, and the muscles of the belly continue moving forward and backward, massaging the organs of the chest and abdominal cavities. Intestinal peristalsis also improves, contributing to better digestion and excretion. In addition, this kind of breathing stimulates the vagus nerve—part of the parasympathetic nervous system, as described in Chapter 2—relaxing the muscles and expanding peripheral blood vessels, facilitating adequate blood supply throughout the body.

We can create a solid energy center in our lower abdomen through breathing. If you inhale and exhale each breath mindfully, focusing on this energy center, your belly will heat up, and hot energy will push the water energy of your kidneys upward to cool your head. Once you're skilled at abdominal breathing, you'll be able to feel your lower dahnjon warming, a pleasant heat radiating from the center of your belly and spreading to your whole abdomen and lower back. Then you will automatically develop Water Up, Fire Down circulation, activating all the vital phenomena of your body.

However, many people have difficulty with abdominal breathing because their Fire Ways are blocked by emotional stress. If they try to breathe with their belly when they're not relaxed, they might end up with an even more stifling, constricting feeling in their chest because their fire energy has reversed course, rising instead of sinking. I've developed a practice to deal with this problem, Joongwan Healing, which I will introduce in Chapter 9. The purpose of Joongwan Healing is to open the blocked Fire Way, releasing emotional energy built up in the chest, and to breathe deeply by relaxing the body. It's good to do plenty of Joongwan Healing before going on to abdominal breathing.

One of the advantages of breathing practice is that you can do it anytime and anywhere—while you're working, while you're eating, even while attending a meeting. Breathing happens automatically even if you don't try to manipulate it, but if you breathe *intentionally*—deeply, slowly, and evenly—it becomes a powerful tool for water-fire energy circulation.

Meditate

Many people used to think of meditation as sitting for hours without budging, wearing unusual clothes, at a temple or ashram deep in the mountains. Now meditation has been popularized so much that you can even sit at your desk in an office to meditate, perhaps using an app on your cell phone as a guide. It's a welcome development that meditation has become "cool," something many want to do, and not the exclusive property of a small minority.

But what is meditation? The core of meditation is turning your outwardly focused consciousness inward, feeling yourself as you are, here and now. As we go about our daily lives, our awareness inevitably turns outward. And our heads are bound to become a complex tangle of thoughts.

Remember what I said in Chapter 5, that cutting off thoughts provides true rest for an overheated brain. Stopping your thinking, though, is no easy task. Right now, close your eyes and try not to think of anything at all for a moment.

Did that go well? More thoughts probably arose in your mind. That's why we need something to anchor our restless minds, which ceaselessly create thoughts and seesaw back and forth from one thought to another.

Let's say you have a curious, active three-year-old. To her, everything is amazing. She wants to touch and put in her mouth everything she sees, toss everything she can lay her hands on, and push everything off the table onto the floor. She wants to follow you wherever you go, even to the bathroom. What do you do, then, to keep your child still? A method used by many parents is to offer her a toy or play a video on the phone.

No different from children, our minds need something like that, too. But what anchors our minds has to be something *inside* us, not a toy or some kind of entertainment. The best thing you can use as an anchor is your own body. Quietly close your eyes and concentrate on your body. Feel your breathing, the sense of energy in your body, its temperature. When you feel the vital phenomena arising in your body, your mind remains in the here and now, not going into the past or the future. This is the best way to put your thoughts to rest.

Quietly focusing on your vital phenomena, you can feel them growing more vigorous. Energy and blood flow better throughout your body—and when energy flows, blockages open up, the cloudy becomes clear, and complicated messes are put in good order. Your thoughts gradually decrease, and your mind grows tranquil. Water Up, Fire Down energy circulation happens automatically, your head cooling and your belly warming.

Now tranquil, your mind won't be perturbed if you hoist its anchor. At first you feel your energy, your breathing, the different sensations in your body, but then you become completely one with what you feel. You become energy itself, breathing itself. You feel a sense of total oneness with yourself. Then you're in a state of true meditation, your thoughts totally silenced and your mind emptied of mental representations.

Exercise

As a way to recover water-fire energy circulation, many people may think only of sitting with their eyes closed, meditating or breathing. But moving your body—especially doing exercises to train your muscles and move your joints—is a very effective method for changing your energy. That's why I consider exercises that actively move the body every bit as important as sitting and quietly concentrating on the body. For those who get sleepy when they sit down to meditate, their heads filling with distracting thoughts, I generally advise that they do basic physical training—especially lots of exercise that works the lower body, which strengthens the lower dahnjon in the belly, stabilizing energy.

Exercise positively affects health in countless ways. Regular exercise strengthens bones, joints, and muscles, and it develops the basic level of fitness we need for our daily lives—muscle strength, lung capacity, balance, quick reflexes, and flexibility. It also enables you to maintain your optimal weight and strengthens your heart and blood vessels, preventing cardiovascular disease.

Exercise is good for the brain, too. Working out increases blood flow to the brain, improving memory and learning ability, and enhancing concentration. It causes the secretion of serotonin and dopamine hormones, which help provide feelings of happiness and well-being, reducing depression and anxiety. The enhanced oxygen supply to the brain helps reduce feelings of fatigue and helplessness and helps make it possible to get good-quality sleep at night.

Moving your body is very effective for resting your brain. It's the easiest thing you can do when you can't break the chain of negative thoughts or your chest feels stifled by emotional energy. For some people, moving is easier than meditating or breathing. When you're stressed out, your head hot and your chest constricted, you may have had the experience of your whole body feeling refreshed after a hot, sweaty workout—perhaps running a lap around the neighborhood or doing weight training at the gym. This feeling of rejuvenation arises because physical exercise activates the discharge of stagnant energy in our bodies.

Several exercises are particularly effective for water-fire circulation. The first is tapping specific energy points on our bodies, which opens blocked energy points so that energy can flow well along the meridians. Second are deep-stretching or yoga movements, which gently lengthen the muscles. Movements that twist and squeeze the body particularly facilitate blood circulation to the extremities. The third type of exercise is strength training, especially exercises to develop the core muscles and the muscles of the lower body.

For good water-fire energy circulation, the abdomen and lower part of the body must be warm. Muscles are like power plants generating heat in our bodies; more than 40 percent of our body heat is created in the muscles. When you do strength-training exercises, your muscles repeatedly contract and relax, producing heat. Warm blood pumped by the heart is spread throughout your body by the movement of the muscles. Core strength training corrects posture and forms pressure in the belly, promoting more efficient blood and energy circulation. The thigh muscles account for some 30 percent of the muscle mass in our bodies. Training the muscles of the lower body also raises basal metabolism, which is very helpful for weight management. One of the most simple and effective ways to train the lower body is to do what the human body was built to do—walk. Instead of sitting behind the computer all day, make a point of getting up to walk around several times a day, and take some longer walks, too.

When you have a great worry or concern, it can be difficult to find the presence of mind to sit quietly, control your breath, and meditate. At such times, move your body. Continuously worrying will eat up your energy, exhausting you and making it harder to escape your troubles. But if you move your body, your mind will stabilize, and your brain activity will increase, enabling you to come up with ideas for seeing your way through difficult situations.

Be Aware

Breathing, meditation, and exercise are all tools for moving your energy and changing your energy state. By using these tools, we can create Water Up, Fire Down circulation—the most stable, healthy energy state. Once energy recovers its normal flow, your mind will be stabilized. There is something you come to realize, though, as you change your energy this way. Just as energy changes the mind, so, too, the *mind changes energy*. Your mind is the ultimate tool for maintaining water-fire flow.

You have probably heard about the placebo effect. This refers to something that can happen when you take a fake medication, one without any medicinal value, thinking it's a real drug. The belief of patients who think they'll get better—their autosuggestions—has even cured such severe diseases as cancer. The placebo effect shows us that our bodies respond to our beliefs, whether or not that information is true.

In a famous experiment conducted in 2003 by neuroscientists at Harvard Medical School, subjects imagined playing the piano for five weeks. They never used an actual instrument, but nonetheless the part of their brains that controls finger movements grew. This shows that the physical structure of the brain can be changed by our imagination alone.

Right now, numerous thoughts and emotions are arising in our minds. And those thoughts and emotions cause a variety of physiological reactions in our bodies. If you think joyful, happy thoughts, your body secretes good hormones, but if you stay too long mired in negative feelings, your body secretes harmful hormones. Just as a flying insect no bigger than your fingertip creates waves as it skips across the surface of a still lake, all thoughts and emotions cause changes in energy. So it's hard to maintain Water Up, Fire Down circulation without controlling your thoughts and emotions.

What state of mind allows good control of thoughts and emotions? It requires a mindset that lets you observe what's happening in the present, calmly watching without judgment or attachment, and without going into the past or the future. This is what is commonly called "mindfulness."

If you watch the thoughts and emotions rising in your mind just as they are—without trying to change or eliminate them and without evaluating them as good or bad—they will gradually subside. The mind that serenely watches the various thoughts and feelings arising within, without being attached to any of them, has the power to return everything to a natural, balanced state. This is central to the meditation I mentioned earlier in this chapter. This attitude creates water-fire energy circulation.

Practice watching your thoughts and emotions arise without getting stuck in them. When you feel anger toward someone, simply observe the feeling, "I'm mad at someone now." If you're ashamed or disgusted with yourself over what you did at work today, just observe, "Self-disgust is rising in me now." Watch the phenomena appearing in your mind the way a calm lake reflects the ever-changing clouds in the sky.

Doing that will open a gap between you and your thoughts or emotions. Space will appear between the two, which had previously seemed inseparable. Then you will be able to objectify your thoughts and emotions or your situation without identifying yourself with them. You'll realize that your thoughts and emotions are not you; they are just phenomena arising in your mind. Then you'll be able to consider your choices dispassionately instead of reacting to your thoughts or feelings.

It's not easy to move a cushion while you're sitting on it. Of course, you could scoot it along with your buttocks, but you can move it much more easily and gracefully by standing and picking it up. In the same way, it's hard to escape from your worries and anxieties while you're clinging to them, but they'll naturally fall away if you take a step back to look at them.

Practice watching everything that is happening, here and now, with detachment—as an observer. Later, you'll also develop a sense for focusing your mind entirely on certain thoughts, emotions, and objects. You'll come to see that by not immediately reacting to thoughts or emotions, but instead watching them dispassionately with your mind, you can make them disappear. You'll find that you can consciously use your mind to create and move thoughts, emotions, and energies.

A mind that observes disinterestedly, without craving or fear, has powerful strength for moving energy. If you focus this mind in your belly, imagining heat, your abdomen will grow hot. If you focus on your chest with this mind, summoning a gentle, compassionate energy embracing all things, your heart will fill with that energy. If you send this mental energy into your brain, imagining cool dew falling upon it, your brain will become cooler. And if this mind concentrates on something you really want to achieve, you will manifest incredible creativity and drive.

We normally focus when there's something in particular that we want to do, but that concentration is bound to include a mixture of tension, expectation, intense ambition, and, at the same time, fear that it may not go well. Yet if we practice observing without attachment or judgment, we can apply unimaginably powerful attention—pristine and pure—without the unwanted distractions of the mind. This detached observation has the power to return everything to a condition of balance and harmony—to its original state of Water Up, Fire Down energy circulation that makes the cycle of life possible.

SUMMARY

- Use four tools to achieve good water-fire balance: breathing, meditation, exercise, and awareness.

- The ideal way to breathe is deeply and slowly into your lower abdomen.

- Meditate by focusing on your body's energy sensations.

- Move your body, including strengthening your muscles and joints, to change your energy.

- Practice detached awareness by observing your thoughts and emotions without judgment.

No matter what physical or mental issues you may have, if you apply the Water Up, Fire Down energy principle in your daily life, you can make progress toward clearing them up.

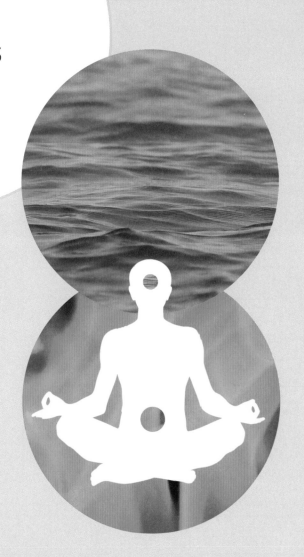

PART 2
Training
Routines

CHAPTER 7

Before You Begin Practice

Simply knowing something in your mind is not enough; true knowledge requires action. Knowing the meaning of the word "honest," for example, doesn't make you honest; only a life lived truthfully will make you an honest person. The same is true for the principle we are examining here. Understanding the principle of Water Up, Fire Down energy flow outlined in this book doesn't give you the perfect energy balance. Rather, it is determined by whether you develop everyday habits that help you stay in good health.

People typically show two patterns of response when I lecture on health: "Oh, who doesn't know that?" and "You're right, but who has the time for that?" If you want a healthy life, drop these two excuses right now. Knowing something isn't what matters. In the end, it's your actions that determine your health. If you value your health, shouldn't you invest time in protecting and developing it?

You don't need to do every training method introduced in this book. But you do need to practice daily the ones that help you, even if just a few of them. Like eating, washing your face, and brushing your teeth every day, make water-fire energy circulation a regular part of your health and fitness routine.

Abandon the Thought That Change Takes a Lot of Time

How much distance is there between happiness and unhappiness? How much time does it take to become unhappy and then happy again? If that's hard to answer, let's change the question: How long does it take you to get angry? No time at all. In the same way, it takes no time at all for your mood to improve. This is simply a function of our minds.

Both happiness and unhappiness are kinds of energy phenomena. Once we realize that we are in a state of unhappy, stifling energy, it's up to us to change our energy. We can continue as we are, or we can create happiness. The important thing is to realize that positive energy comes from within us. Instead of waiting for others to make you happy or for good fortune to come your way, you can make yourself happy right now. Realize that ultimately, it comes from within yourself, and happiness starts with the choice to be happy. Then, make the choices that help you in that direction. Listening to music, eating fresh fruit, going for a walk and enjoying the fresh air—immediate actions like these, though seemingly trivial, can give you a definite taste of happiness.

This goes for health and healing as well. It doesn't take a lot of time to switch from an unhealthy energy state to a healthy one. As soon as you act, your energy starts to change, and transformations appear. Of course, it may take considerable time for long-standing diseases to heal completely.

Changes happen now if you act now. That is a law of energy:

"Where the mind goes, energy follows."

If you continue changing your energy in this way, your health will definitely improve since both health and disease are energy phenomena. If your body feels stiff and achy, your chest feels stuffy, and you're in a bad mood, instead of staying in that condition, you can change your energy immediately using the methods of Water Up, Fire Down circulation I will introduce in this book.

Interact with Your Brain as You Practice

When you do these exercises, connect with both your brain and your body. Make sure that your brain recognizes the changes you feel in your body. Help your brain scan your condition and recognize the subtle changes in your body's senses. Here are a few things that people commonly notice during or after exercise:

> *"My head is hot and foggy."*
>
> *"My eyes are dry and blurry."*
>
> *"My chest feels tight, like it's totally blocked."*
>
> *"My neck and shoulders are stiff."*
>
> *"I feel pain when I press my Fire Way."*
>
> *"My belly and legs feel cold."*
>
> *"After tapping my belly, I keep burping."*
>
> *"After training, my mouth fills with saliva, my eyes are moist, my hands and feet are warmer, and my breathing is much more comfortable."*

Your experience may be like some of these or something entirely different. Whatever happens, watch carefully and express what you observe concretely to let your brain recognize changes in your physical condition and senses.

When it recognizes discomfort in your body, your brain starts actively working to solve the problem. This natural healing power is latent in everyone's brains and bodies. It is not something artificial; it's a blessing that nature has given all of us. Let your brain know that you want to be healthy and that you're interested in the state of your body. Your brain will definitely respond.

Check the State of Your Water-Fire Circulation

When our bodies have good water-fire flow, the energy center in our guts is warm and filled with vital energy. The energy center in our chests then opens, feeling lighter and less congested, and the energy center in our heads becomes cooler and clearer. In short, a warm belly, open heart, and cool head have been reestablished— our body's ideal energy state. Broken water-fire energy balance, on the other hand, leads to declining health in the body's three energy centers, causing various physical, emotional, and mental problems.

The following questions will help you check your water-fire energy balance. See how many you can answer yes to.

- ☐ Does your head feel heavy and cloudy, and do you have frequent headaches?

- ☐ Are your eyes often blurry and dry?

- ☐ Are your mouth and throat frequently dry?

- ☐ Are your shoulders stiff, and your face and neck often hot?

- ☐ Do you have a stifling feeling in your chest, and is your breathing uncomfortable?

- ☐ Is your belly often cold?

- ☐ Do you have frequent indigestion and bloating?

- ☐ Are your hands and feet cold or frequently numb?

- ☐ Are you always tired and have trouble recovering your energy, even with rest?

- ☐ Are your joints often painful and stiff?

- ☐ Do you have trouble getting to sleep at night?

- ☐ Do you get anxious or irritated easily?

- ☐ Once you start worrying, is it not easy to stop?

- ☐ Do you often feel resentful and angry?

- ☐ Do you feel depressed and lack self-esteem?

If you answered yes to 0 to 4 of these questions, your body's energy is in a relatively well-circulated and balanced state. Based on your core's vital energy, your motivation, and your positive mind, you seem to be building a healthy and vibrant life in your own way. But stay vigilant and continue to care for your health. Hopefully your energy center will be further strengthened, making it as strong and stable as a pillar that will not sway in any change.

If you answered yes to 5 to 9 of these questions, then pay more attention to your energy state. These symptoms suggest that your energy is easily affected by changes in any event, environment, or information you experience. To stabilize your condition, focus on developing your energy centers, strengthening your core, and opening your chest.

If you answered yes to 10 or more, your energy circulation is considerably reduced, and you're in a dangerous state of unbalanced energy. Since energy is very unstable in such a situation, you may experience intense fluctuations in your emotions and attitudes toward life. If your situation is even more severe, you may find yourself feeling helpless and desperate. Start by strengthening the energy of your core to prevent further imbalance.

CHAPTER 8

Keep Your Belly Warm

W hen your head feels overheated—when you realize that you're no longer in good water-fire energy flow, your head no longer cool and your belly no longer warm— remember this one thing: no matter what, you have to make the heat in your head go down.

What should you do to move the heat down? It's simple—just exercise your lower body. Moving and stimulating your lower body naturally activates the energy in your core, generating heat. When heat is generated in the lower body, the upper body and head do the opposite—they cool down.

Before doing exercises for strengthening your lower body and core, check the current condition of your core energy. This will let you feel how your energy changes after you do the exercises.

Before You Begin: Check Your Core Energy

1. Does your lower belly feel warm?

With your eyes closed and your mind focused on your lower belly, try to feel the temperature there. Does it feel warm, or is it lukewarm or cold? Now focus on your legs and feet and try to feel the temperature there. Do they feel warm, or lukewarm or cold? It's important to feel whether the energy within is hot or cold, not the temperature of the skin's surface. Concentrate one by one on your abdomen, buttocks, lower back, thighs, calves, and feet, trying to feel their temperatures.

2. How deep is your breathing?

When you inhale, check how deep the breath comes into your body—whether it reaches your chest, diaphragm, or lower abdomen. First place one hand on your chest and the other hand on your upper abdomen. If your chest moves more when you breathe, the breath is coming in as far as your chest, and if your upper abdomen moves more, it's reaching your diaphragm. Now place one hand on your upper abdomen and the other below your navel. If your lower belly moves more, your breathing is coming deep into your lower abdomen. Try to feel whether your breathing is long and smooth, or short and rough.

3. How is the movement of your abdomen and intestines?

Observe whether your breathing goes deeply into the abdomen. If your breathing goes deep into your lower belly, your abdomen will naturally expand and contract as your breath comes in and out. If your abdomen and intestines move very little or not at all, you have what I call "a stiff gut." You can check for places where your gut feels stiff or painful by bringing the fingers of both hands together and pressing deeply into every part of your abdomen in succession. Start from the center of your upper abdomen and press around your abdomen in a clockwise circle.

TAP YOUR BELLY

The most direct method of activating your core energy is to physically stimulate your belly. All you have to do is use your hands to tap your lower dahnjon, the energy center of your core. This is called Dahnjon Tapping.

DAHNJON TAPPING

1. Stand with your feet shoulder-width apart and bend your knees slightly. Tuck your chin a little, close your eyes, and focus your mind on your lower abdomen.

2. *Dahnjon Tapping Method 1:* Tap your belly using the lower part of your loose fists, where your little fingers are located. Alternating hands, tap rapidly with enough force to stimulate your belly.

3. *Dahnjon Tapping Method 2:* Tap your lower abdomen using both open palms at the same time. Thinking of your lower abdomen as a drum, beat it with your hands in a steady rhythm. Use enough force to make a sound.

4. Do Dahnjon Tapping using both methods, for as few as 100 to as many as 500 or even 1,000 repetitions. It takes less than a minute to tap 100 times. Beginners can do about 100 repetitions in a set and then gradually increase that number when they're more familiar with the exercise. It's also okay to take a short break between sets of 100.

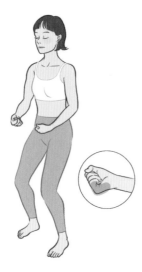
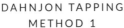
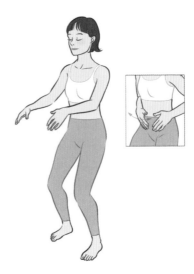

**DAHNJON TAPPING
METHOD 1**

**DAHNJON TAPPING
METHOD 2**

Tip: Relax your upper body when you tap so that your arms and shoulders don't get tense. Slightly bending your knees lowers your center of gravity into your lower body, letting you relax your upper body as you exercise comfortably.

After Exercising: With your knees slightly bent and your palms placed over your lower belly, close your eyes and focus on your abdomen, trying to feel your breathing and gut. How far in do your breaths go? Do you feel your gut moving, your belly expanding and contracting as you breathe? As energy collects there, try to feel your belly gradually growing warmer.

EXERCISE YOUR GUT

After doing Dahnjon Tapping, you probably noticed that the movement of your gut is coordinated with your breathing. As your belly expands and contracts with the coming and going of your breath, your intestines move naturally, and your breaths sink deep into your abdomen. Thus, if your gut is moving well, you know that your breathing is deep and stable. If it's not, your breathing is shallow and unstable.

You can begin to improve the depth of your breathing by first loosening up your intestines. The following two exercises are especially effective for releasing tension from the abdomen. And since one-third of the body's total blood volume circulates through the gut, these exercises also help with blood circulation throughout the body, lessening the burden on the heart.

INTESTINAL EXERCISE

When doing this exercise, you don't necessarily have to sync your breathing with your intestinal movements. Just concentrating on the exercise will naturally lead to deeper breathing.

1. Stand with your feet shoulder-width apart and bend your knees slightly. Tuck your chin a little, close your eyes, and focus your mind inside your lower abdomen.

2. Place your palms on your lower belly with your thumbs at your navel and your index fingers touching, as shown in the following figure.

3. Pull your abdomen in toward your back, hold it for a moment, and then relax, releasing your belly naturally.

4. Repeat 100 times, pulling and releasing your abdomen. Increase the number of repetitions as you become more comfortable with the exercise.

5. Once you're comfortable with the exercise, pull your belly more strongly toward your back as you do it.

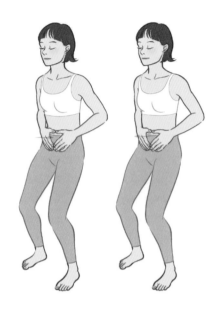

Tip: When doing Intestinal Exercise for the first time, some people may feel pain in their abdomen or lower back if their gut is stiff. If this applies to you, use your palm to massage these spots and release the stiffness, then gently resume doing Intestinal Exercise without being too intense. Also, relax when doing the exercise so that your arms and shoulders don't become tense.

INTESTINAL EXERCISE USING A TOOL

The benefits of Intestinal Exercise can be accentuated using a tool I call a Belly Button Healing Wand. It's quite effective, especially for beginners and for those whose guts are particularly stiff. It's also perfectly fine to use any sort of blunt stick instead.

1.   Adopt the same posture as before for the Intestinal Exercise.

2.   Place the tip of the Belly Button Healing Wand or stick against your abdomen, about two inches below your navel. Press the tool in and then release it. Do this rhythmically and at the relatively fast pace of about 120 repetitions per minute. I describe this as "pumping." Using a tool makes it much easier to exercise your lower belly. Pump your lower abdomen about 200 to 300 times.

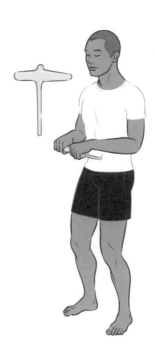

3.   Now place the end of the tool against your navel and pump your belly button 200 to 300 times, using the same method as above. I call this technique "Belly Button Healing." This way you can effectively exercise your entire gut and abdominal muscles through your navel at the very center of your abdomen.

Tip: When pumping your lower abdomen and belly button, place the tool over clothing, not on your bare skin. If you're lying down, it's a good idea to place a towel as a buffer on the spot where you'll be pumping. You can refer to my book *Belly Button Healing* for more details on the principles and effects of this practice.

After Exercising: Set down the tool and place your palms on your lower abdomen, bending your knees slightly. Close your eyes and concentrate on your lower abdomen, trying to feel your breathing and your guts moving. Your breathing will feel much more robust and deeper in your abdomen now, your intestines moving much more than when you did the exercise without the tool.

TRAIN YOUR LOWER BODY

One effective way to increase your core temperature is to work out your lower body. Muscles generate more than 40 percent of the body's heat, and 70 percent of all muscles are in the lower body. The easiest exercise to move the heat down and increase your core temperature is one you probably already do every day—walking.

More than just your leg muscles are exercised when you walk. The motion of moving your legs back and forth works the muscles surrounding your core and the iliopsoas muscle connecting your lower back, pelvis, and thighs. This automatically trains your abdominal organs, making it possible for your breathing to sink deep into your abdomen.

You've probably felt your temperature rising after walking, especially in your feet. The temperature of your feet increases because every step you take stimulates your soles. This action creates an energy state in which the head is cooler and the feet are warmer.

POWER WALKING

The most effective way of walking for your lower body and core is power walking. This means fast and forceful walking, not taking your time as if out for a stroll.

1. Walk faster and more forcefully than usual.

2. Keep your upper body straight and step with heels first, extending your legs as far as you can.

3. It's okay to lower your arms to your sides, but you'll put more power in your steps if you bend them, moving them forward and backward as you walk.

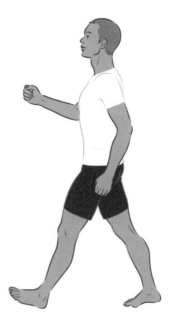

4. Amplify the effectiveness by making your strides longer than normal.

5. Tighten the muscles of your waist and belly as you walk, sensing that your muscles, pelvis, and gut are being worked with every step.

Walking for an hour a day is great, but try to walk at least 20 to 30 minutes every day. Try walking right now, noticing how your core grows warmer. Then check the energy state of your body. You'll be able to feel definite changes.

Tip: Walk outdoors if possible. If that's not possible, any form of walking will do. Even walking in place exercises your lower body, activating and circulating your core energy. Squats are also highly effective since they work the muscles of the thighs and buttocks in a focused way.

After Exercising: Focus your mind on your belly and lower body, trying to feel the temperature there. Do you feel heaviness, tingling, or other energy sensations? Do you feel your temperature rising or your feet growing warmer?

Try to feel whether your breathing is coming into your abdomen deeper and stronger than before. How about the movement of your gut, along with your breathing? Observe whether your abdomen expands and contracts naturally with your breath going in and out.

CHAPTER 9

Open Your Blocked Chest

To make the heat in your head descend into your gut, you must open up your Fire Way, the energy path between your head and your abdomen. Energy stagnation in your chest keeps the heat in your head from sinking into your belly—commonly described as "having a blockage in the chest." Just as traffic won't flow smoothly after a freeway accident if cars are blocking the middle of the road, stagnated energy in your chest keeps fire energy from sinking down your Fire Way.

But how do you open your chest if it is blocked? You must activate the energy center in your middle dahnjon, also known as the "heart chakra." Discharge the heavy, cloudy energy festering there and allow light, clear energy to circulate instead.

Heavy, dark energy generally comes from negative emotions we have held onto for a long time. Our bodies and minds are energy, and so are our feelings. The energy of negative emotions—anger, resentment, depression, anxiety, nervousness, irritation, sadness, shame, victim consciousness, arrogance—accumulates in our conscious and unconscious minds, forming energetic lumps in our hearts. The degree to which this happens differs from person to person, but it affects most of us since we are all being exposed to more stress and emotional upset than ever before.

If unresolved, negative energy will continue to block the chest, and heat will accumulate in the head and the chest because it can't descend smoothly into the abdomen. And the abdomen can't heat up because, with the chest blocked, fire energy can't descend deep into the belly with breathing.

Before You Begin: Check the Energy Balance of Your Chest

Before you begin doing the exercises that follow, use the following checklist to examine the state of energy in your chest.

1. Does your chest feel tight or stuffy?

Have you ever felt that your chest was tight or stuffy? You might not have noticed it in your ordinary daily life, but close your eyes now and try to focus on your chest. Do you get the feeling that your chest is comfortable and wide open? Or does it feel constricted and stifled? If you tend to be dominated by negative emotions like stress, anger, anxiety, and worry, the energy of those feelings may be stuck in your chest.

2. How deep and comfortable is your breathing?

Ideally your chest should have a wide-open, comfortable feeling. You can check the state of energy in your chest right now if you examine your breathing. Close your eyes and focus on your chest, trying to sense the character of your breathing. Is it comfortable and deep, or shallow and rapid? If your breathing is comfortable—deep, smooth, and natural, with nothing hindering it—then you're in a state of good water-fire circulation. But if your breaths are uneven and short and your breathing is uncomfortable, your chest is blocked by something.

3. How intense is the pain when you press the center of your chest?

You can actually check your chest condition by touch, as I described in Chapter 5. With your thumb, press hard on the center of your sternum—your middle dahnjon energy point. Then rub that spot in a circle two or three times. How intense is the pain you feel? If you gradually go up along the centerline of your chest, pressing different spots up to the base of your throat, you will discover places where the pain feels more intense. Look on the pain as a reflection of how much stress you're under and as a sign that you have blockages in your chest.

OPENING BLOCKAGES CAUSED BY WORRY AND ANXIETY

There are many ways to open your Fire Way. One of these is Joongwan Healing, a method of self-healing I developed recently. Joongwan Healing is highly effective for relaxing a tense body and mind and for discharging emotional energy—stress, worry, anxiety, nervousness, and depression—that has built up over time. This exercise is not difficult at all, so be sure to give it a try. Let's start by looking at why healing the Joongwan point is essential, how Joongwan Healing works, and what effects it has.

Open Your Joongwan, a Zone of Fire-Energy Stagnation

There are a few places on the Fire Way where energy is easily blocked and an energy bottleneck develops. One of these is the energy point called the *Joongwan*, located in the middle of the upper abdomen. With your thumb touching the point where the left and right sides of your ribs converge and your ring finger touching your belly button, gently bend your index finger inward until it touches the midline of your body. The point that the tip of your index finger touches is your Joongwan.

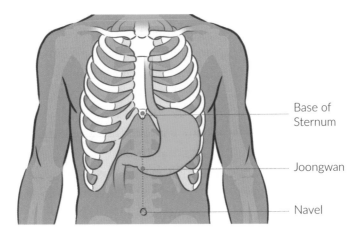

Base of
Sternum

Joongwan

Navel

LOCATION OF THE JOONGWAN POINT

The area from the bottom of your sternum to your belly button is your upper abdomen, and the area below your belly button is your lower abdomen. The Joongwan is the energy point in the very middle of your upper abdomen. Joongwan, in fact, means "center of the stomach." Generally, it is close to the pylorus, which is where the stomach leads into the small intestine, although its precise location can differ from person to person. The Joongwan is one of the most important energy control centers in the body.

Almost all the digestive organs—including the stomach, liver, gallbladder, and upper parts of the intestines—are in the upper abdomen. In traditional Asian medicine, the Joongwan is considered to be the starting point for energy circulation through the body's organs, as well as the place where energy returns after finishing its cycle through the body. It's most directly related to the stomach but also has a crucial effect on other organs.

Various digestive disorders appear when the Joongwan is blocked. The most common is uncomfortable bloating caused by indigestion. Other typical symptoms include abdominal pain, diarrhea, constipation, intestinal inflammation, reflux esophagitis, and problems of the spleen and pancreas. When such symptoms are present, traditional Asian medicine treats them by using acupuncture or moxibustion on the Joongwan.

The stomach is especially important because it is your body's energy power plant. In addition to being an important energy center, the stomach digests food and absorbs nutrients to be turned into energy. Consequently, when your Joongwan is blocked so your stomach doesn't have enough energy or energy flow, you develop digestive disorders and you feel weak, even when you've had plenty to eat. Also, you lack ambition and often feel fatigued.

You may also be aware that your digestive organs are intimately connected with your emotions. When you're tense or stressed before a presentation you have to make, you may experience nausea and indigestion. When you feel fear or nervousness, your guts stiffen and contract, giving you that "butterflies in the stomach" feeling. You also may have noticed that you go to the bathroom frequently when you're in a bad mood or tense. Or you may have a craving for a certain "comfort food" when you're stressed out. Why is it that our stomachs are so tuned in to our emotions?

According to scientists, this phenomenon happens because of our "gut-brain" and intestinal microorganisms. Hundreds of millions of nerve cells are distributed along the intestinal wall, which together act somewhat independently of the brain in our heads. That is why this system of neurons is called the gut-brain. Our intestines contain more microbes than there are human cells in our bodies. These microorganisms are involved in regulating intestinal motility and immune response, and they make a variety of hormones and neurotransmitters that affect our brains and bodies.

Neurotransmitters associated with joy, happiness, and tranquility—including dopamine, serotonin, and GABA—are made by intestinal microbes and cells in the intestinal walls, as well as by our brains. Our brains, gut-brains, and microorganisms exchange biological information through the information highway called the "gut-brain axis." Thus, the condition of one area affects the condition of the other. For example, being in a bad mood makes your stomach hurt, and a stomachache puts you in a bad mood.

Because of this correlation between your guts and your emotions, stimulating your Joongwan point can improve both the physical function of your digestive organs and your mental health, easing anxiety, nervousness, and depression. Emotional stability returns as the once-blocked Joongwan opens and fire energy that had stagnated in the Fire Way sinks into the abdomen, restoring water-fire energy balance.

Rapid Relaxation and Better Mood through Joongwan Healing

Joongwan Healing involves repeatedly pressing your Joongwan point using either your hand or a tool. It includes two exercises: Joongwan Pumping, rapidly and rhythmically pressing the Joongwan, and Joongwan Breathing, slowly and gently pressing the Joongwan while breathing. The abdominal aorta passes below the Joongwan point, and Joongwan Healing helps it contract and expand repeatedly. This quickly helps improve the energy and blood circulation of the whole body. And by expanding your chest cavity to breathe in as much air as possible, you can supply a great deal of oxygen to your body.

Joongwan Healing practitioners commonly experience a number

of positive effects. First, it improves digestive function. Joongwan Healing physically moves the intestines, producing burping and rumbling in the gut. Tightness and bloating is reduced, and the stomach becomes more comfortable. People who spend a lot of time in the bathroom because of diarrhea or constipation often return to normal right away. Reduction in reflux esophagitis, a condition causing heartburn after eating, is also commonly reported.

Second, Joongwan Healing relieves tension, relaxing the body and calming the mind. People with considerable blockage in their Joongwan may feel pain or tension in the area of this energy point, or they may even feel nauseated when they begin the practice. The discomfort disappears for most, though, if they keep at it. The muscles of the face, shoulders, chest, and middle back relax, and anxiety and nervousness diminish. Sometimes for the first time in a long time, they're able to get to sleep and enjoy a good night's rest.

Third, practitioners are able to breathe deeply. Even those with shallow, fast, rough breathing find that their breathing is consistently deeper, slower, and smoother after doing Joongwan Healing. They have the feeling that their breath suddenly goes deep into their lower belly. For those accustomed to abdominal breathing, as discussed in Chapter 6, doing so after Joongwan Healing causes their breath to fill completely from the lower to the upper abdomen, letting them feel like they are breathing with their whole trunk.

Fourth, the body becomes warmer. With Joongwan Healing, the hands and feet get warmer, as do the belly and back. The effects can be felt very distinctly after just a few minutes of Joongwan Healing. The whole body feels so much warmer that beads of sweat may stand out on the forehead. This is likely due to more vigorous blood circulation, an effect of deep, stable breathing, relaxation and contraction of the abdominal aorta, and intestinal massage.

Also frequently reported are clearer and lighter heads; posture improved by relaxation of the upper back, shoulders, and chest; moister, brighter eyes; and saliva pooling in the mouth. All these physiological phenomena appear when we develop Water Up, Fire Down energy circulation.

Among the effects frequently shared by those who practice Joongwan Healing is something especially noteworthy: "I can now notice the tension in my body better." People end up more actively recognizing and resolving stress, they say, because being under stress feels like lumps building up and blocking the Joongwan area. Once in the habit of stuffing herself with food when stressed, one individual said that a little over a month after beginning Joongwan Healing, she started feeling her Joongwan getting blocked when she overate. That was uncomfortable, so she became better able to control her eating.

These are all phenomena of Water Up, Fire Down energy circulation, developments that appear when our bodies recover their sense for achieving harmony and balance.

Without Self-Love, the Joongwan Is Blocked

According to the yogic philosophy of India, our bodies have seven energy centers, called chakras. Each chakra has a specific role related to our physical, mental, and spiritual development. The Joongwan is the site of the third of these chakras, the solar plexus chakra, which is associated with personal identity and personal power. Whether you have a healthy or distorted self-image depends on the condition of this chakra.

When the energy of the solar plexus is healthy and harmonious, it manifests in a personality as self-respect, self-acceptance, and self-confidence. You express your feelings and thoughts with confidence and take responsibility for your words and deeds. You have the power to put your choices into action. "This is my life. I can direct my life as I want. I love myself and my life." Basically, if your solar plexus functions well, you live your life with confidence and a positive attitude. You also have healthy boundaries with the people around you, treating them fairly, not criticizing or judging others.

When the energy of your solar plexus is not harmonious, it manifests as excessive self-display, arrogance, and a desire to control others. You may become a strict perfectionist, critical and intolerant of other people. And if the energy of this chakra is too weak, you get stuck in self-contempt and feelings of inferiority. You come to have a miserable self-image, worrying about what others think and hiding your feelings and thoughts to get their approval. Unhappy with yourself and often misunderstanding the intentions of other people, you easily get stuck in victim consciousness.

The character this chakra expresses isn't set in stone. As we learn through our life experiences, we continue developing each of our chakras. The nature of the solar plexus chakra is not fixed, either. Sometimes we like and are honest with ourselves, coolly accepting our mistakes, and we can dispassionately take feedback about ourselves from other people. At other times, though, we dislike ourselves. We criticize or flatter others to protect ourselves, and we feel pathetic if other people don't give us recognition. In other words, our thoughts and even our personalities change, depending on the state of our energy.

Joongwan and *solar plexus chakra* are different names for the same energy center. The psychological function of this energy center is to establish your relationship with yourself. You can have good relationships with other people only when you have a good relationship with yourself. Most importantly, you must have respect and love for yourself.

Respecting yourself means having basic trust in yourself. People who respect themselves don't disparage themselves when faced with a challenge or when things don't go their way. They also have healthy boundaries when they deal with family, friends, colleagues, and others. When you have respect and affection for yourself, you can express yourself openly, being honest about what you want or need. Your relationships with others become smooth once you've formed a good relationship with yourself.

To have a healthy body and mind, you need an underlying foundation of self-respect. This means taking an interest in your body and striving to take care of your health because you love and respect yourself. Without self-respect, mottos such as "My health, my responsibility" are powerless. Without self-respect you lack confidence, so you have no certainty when it comes to your own choices. Even after making decisions, you're unable to push forward with drive, or you feel burdened when taking responsibility for your choices. And you become dependent on others because you're afraid you may be left alone or may not receive enough recognition and love.

Of the two energy states—good water-fire flow and reversed water-fire flow—which one would help you form a better relationship with yourself, letting you respect and love yourself? It's the state of good water-fire energy, of course.

Given our modern lifestyles—our bodies and minds tense, surrounded by endless competition and judgment—a conscious effort is required to avoid remaining in a state of reversed water-fire circulation for too long. If your Fire Way is blocked, you live with fire energy in your chest, which sparks an upward blaze of fire energy when even trivial stressors arise. And you grow anxious for no special reason because fire energy continues to roil in your chest. When you're always anxious and ready to burst out in anger, it's hard to establish a healthy self. Opening your blocked Fire Way and regaining good water-fire energy circulation not only allows you to have good health but also lets you recover the trust in and love for yourself that is essential for facing life's challenges with strength and courage. I often say that Joongwan Healing is a breathing practice that creates a physiological and energetic base for loving ourselves. And since it makes our frustrated, heavy hearts brighter and lighter, I've also called it the "Get Bright Method."

How to Do Joongwan Healing

You can do Joongwan Healing using your hands or a tool such as the Belly Button Healing Wand that I introduced in Chapter 8 for Intestinal Exercise. Before doing Joongwan Healing, first confirm the location of your Joongwan. The exact position is the middle point between your belly button and the place at the bottom of your sternum where your rib cage divides.

You can do this exercise while standing or while sitting on the floor or in a chair. If standing, spread your feet about the width of your shoulders and bend your knees slightly. If you're a beginner, it's a good idea to do Joongwan Healing lying down. The effect is accentuated while lying down because your abdominal muscles can relax more effectively in a horizontal position. You can switch to a sitting or standing posture once you've become more comfortable with the exercise.

Exhaling through your mouth while doing Joongwan Healing will help alleviate any pain you might feel.

JOONGWAN HEALING USING YOUR HANDS

1. Start by doing Joongwan Pumping. Place the index, middle, and ring fingers of both hands over your Joongwan, as shown in the figure. Flexing your fingers, rhythmically and repeatedly press your Joongwan. Pump your hands somewhat rapidly, opening your mouth slightly and exhaling through it. Do about 100 to 200 repetitions.

2. Now we'll do Joongwan Breathing. Pressing deep into your Joongwan with your fingers as you exhale, hold your breath for about five seconds, maintaining the pressure with your hands. Be sure to press more deeply than you'd normally think to do. Now relax your fingers and breathe in deeply. Hold your breath for about five seconds. Continue for 10 to 20 repetitions.

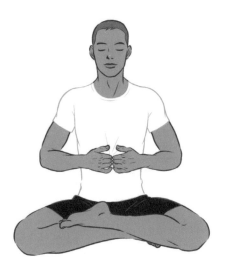

JOONGWAN HEALING USING A TOOL

1. Start by pumping your Joongwan using a Belly Button Healing Wand or a blunt stick. Place the tip of the tool against your Joongwan. Just as you pumped for Intestinal Exercise (Chapter 8), repeatedly pump at a somewhat rapid pace for 100 to 200 repetitions.

2. Now do Joongwan Breathing. Press your Joongwan with your stick or one of the three rods of the Belly Button Healing Wand; it's okay to use the thinnest one, but you can stimulate the point more deeply if you use one of the thicker rods. Pushing the tool in toward your back as you exhale, hold your breath for about five seconds. Inhale deeply, relaxing your hands, and hold for another five seconds. Do 10 to 20 repetitions.

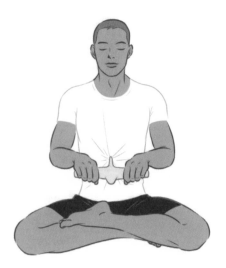

Tip: Take a break if you are feeling uncomfortable, and adjust the intensity of the pressure and repetitions accordingly. When you press in on the exhale, press only until you feel a pulse beating in your abdomen or a slight pain. Take care not to press too hard. Many people experience burping during Joongwan Healing, which is completely normal.

After Exercising: Place your palms on your Joongwan, one over the other. Imagine healing energy coming from your palms and making your Joongwan more comfortable. Breathe in this position for a few minutes without trying to control it. Calmly observe the changes in your body. Do you get the feeling that the energy clogging up your Joongwan is being released?

Pent-up emotional energy is released when you do Joongwan Healing, so this may be hard emotionally. Try to have an attitude of accepting and observing your condition as it is rather than denying or avoiding it. Only then will your emotional pain be healed.

RELEASE THE STRESS IN YOUR CHEST

As I've mentioned, negative emotional energy builds up unconsciously in our hearts, including emotions such as anger, depression, anxiety, nervousness, sadness, shame, victim consciousness, and bigotry. To maintain peace of mind, such emotions and the stress that develops should be resolved as they come up, but many of us just go on as we are, unable to do this. Then the energy of stress and emotion stagnating in the chest prevents fire energy in the head and heart from sinking into the abdomen. This leads to rapid, uncomfortable breathing and an unstable emotional state. Chest Tapping is a way to release stress in the chest.

CHEST TAPPING

1. Sit on the floor or in a chair, straightening your lower back.

2. Tap the left side of your chest with your right fist, using the side of your hand leading into the thumb, as shown in the figure. Closing your eyes and feeling the energy state of your chest, spend about three minutes tapping your chest, including the area below your left collarbone. Tap somewhat forcefully, exhaling through your mouth. Imagine the stagnated energy of stress and emotions being discharged from your chest with your outgoing breath.

3. Switch hands now and tap the right side of your chest with your left hand for about three minutes.

4. Now use whichever hand feels more comfortable and tap along the centerline of your body where your Fire Way passes, including the center of your sternum. Let out the sound, "Ah . . . ," exhaling as you tap, to most effectively discharge stress. Think of yourself as completely releasing all the stress and emotional energy that has been stagnating in your chest.

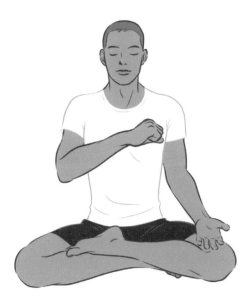

Tip: When you tap your chest for a while, memories of when you've been under stress may come to mind, or the energy of emotions such as anger, sadness, and resentment may come up. You may even feel pity for yourself and regret for having lived with your stress and emotions suppressed instead of resolving them. Release all those energies through your mouth, exhaling with a sound, "Ah . . . ." You may have to repeat this exercise many times for your chest to become really comfortable, depending on how much stress has stagnated and how deeply it is rooted in your energy. Remember—only *you* can heal yourself.

After Exercising: Place your hands on your knees, palms up, and close your eyes. With your mouth slightly open, exhale for a time, "Hoo . . . ," to discharge the stagnant energy from your chest. Now, with your mouth closed, focus your mind on your chest and try to get a sense of the feeling there, the state of energy. Observe whether there is less stress and blockage, whether your chest feels more comfortable or the stifling feeling remains, and whether your breathing is more comfortable and natural.

SEND HEALING ENERGY TO YOUR CHEST

I recommend doing this exercise immediately after the Chest Tapping introduced before. Then, as you gain deeper experience, you'll be able to feel a greater effect.

Our whole bodies are made up of energy, but our hands are where it's easiest to send and receive energy because they have more sense receptors than any other part of the body. You may have also heard about healing therapies using wavelengths of energy emitted from the hands.

Remember the principle that the mind creates energy. Energy goes where you focus your mind. With the certainty that your hands are the greatest healing tools, use them to send healing energy into your weary, troubled heart. Even beginners may experience amazing energy phenomena as well as a more comfortable-feeling chest when they earnestly focus mind and heart on this exercise.

ENERGY HEALING FOR THE CHEST

1. Sit in a chair or in a half-lotus posture on the floor, straightening your lower back.

2. To activate the energy in the palms of your hands, rub your palms together very quickly for 10 to 20 seconds.

3. Hold your palms in front of you so they face each other, leaving about two inches between them. Close your eyes and try to feel the sensations in your hands. You may get a sense of heat or a tingling feeling, which means that energy is being activated. Continue to focus your mind on your hands, imagining healing energy gradually being activated within them.

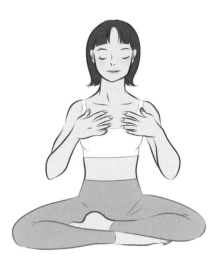

4. Now close your eyes and bring your palms slowly in front of your chest, as shown in the figure. Leave two to three inches of space between your palms and your chest.

5. Visualize warm, healing energy being emitted from your hands and entering your chest.

6. Imagine the healing energy from your hands slowly melting away the heavy emotional baggage that has been

troubling you and making you lonely. In your mind, let go of all the things that you have unconsciously accumulated and clung to.

7. Comfort your heart, saying to it, "You've had a hard time, haven't you? I'm sorry. Don't worry anymore, for I can heal you. I won't trouble you any longer."

8. Feel the healing energy rising in your chest, soaking your heart as if with warm water. As this healing energy is gradually injected into your chest, self-love and esteem are expanding and filling you like air filling a balloon. If you've naturally felt love and gratitude in your heart when doing this exercise, it's a signal that the energy of your middle dahnjon has been healed.

Tip: As with Chest Tapping, pent-up negative emotions may float to the surface even when you send healing energy into your chest. But the more you self-censor when attitudes such as anger, shame, and regret come up—"This isn't good, I should be free of these feelings"—the less you'll be able to resolve them. If you honestly accept yourself—recognizing that you do feel those emotions—and send healing energy into your heart, then the dense energy created by emotional baggage will clear up. You'll be able to feel your emotions losing their hold on you.

CHAPTER 10

Cool Your Overheated Brain

The main reason your brain overheats is that you overuse it. When you focus excessively on something or are lost in endless worry, your brain has to keep working without rest. It is overloaded, so hot energy inevitably rushes in. As your head heats up, it grows heavy, and your mind loses clarity; you might even develop a pounding headache. It's similar to the way a machine or computer overheats if you never let it rest.

Just as our bodies need to rest when they are tired from over-exertion, rest is essential for our overheated brains. That means letting go of your focus and refreshing your brain. If you turn off the power when a machine overheats, it will gradually cool down and return to a normal working state. In the same way, letting your brain cool down allows it to return to its normal energy state. When you focus on work again after your head has cooled, you'll exhibit enhanced powers of concentration. But continuing to work with an overheated brain is not only unproductive, but it will also ruin your health and increase your stress.

We regularly check a machine to make sure it's in good operating condition. Shouldn't we do the same for our bodies, which are far more sensitive than any human-made contraption? Just as there's a standard for what's normal for a machine, so there is for our brains; what's normal is a *cool brain*, not a hot brain. If you maintain this cool state, you'll keep your energy in top shape. *Always* keeping our heads cool isn't easy in our frequently stressed lives, but at the very least we should develop habits that let us detect when our brains are overheated so we can cool them down.

As the master of your own brain, you need to take care of it, just as an equipment manager takes care of machinery. Not detecting or caring whether your brain is overheated is neglecting your responsibilities. Don't be negligent in monitoring your energy state— always remember that you are the master of your brain and your body, as well as their manager.

Before You Begin: Check the Energy Balance of Your Head

1. Is your head hot?

The best way to know if your brain is overheated is to check the temperature of your head. Touch your hand to your forehead right now and try to sense its temperature. You're in top condition if your forehead is cooler than your hand. You can especially feel this condition right after you've woken up from a good, pleasant sleep. Your brain cools down while you sleep because you aren't consciously using it.

If the temperature of your forehead is similar to or just slightly higher than that of your hand, you're still in decent condition. A serious condition is evident when your forehead feels much hotter than your hand.

2. Is your head heavy, and does it ache?

Does your head feel clear and refreshed, or heavy and throbbing? When fire energy rushes to your head, you get the feeling that some kind of heaviness is filling your brain. However, your head should be bright and clear—like a cloudless, azure sky. That's a normal energy condition. The feeling of heavy, murky energy filling your brain like dark clouds is a sign that you need to quickly get out of that condition. Concentration necessarily declines in such a state. Such symptoms commonly appear when not enough oxygen and fresh energy are supplied to the brain through deep, stable breathing.

3. Are your eyes blurry, and is your mouth dry?

The eyes could be seen as the part of the brain that sticks outside the skull. If the brain overheats, the eyes are also affected, becoming dry and making vision blurry. Dry mouth is also evidence that the brain has overheated. In a normal energy state, the eyes are moist and clear, the mouth filled with sweet saliva. But the eyes and mouth can't help but dry out when hot fire energy has risen to the head. If you pay attention in your everyday life, observing whether your eyes and mouth are moist or dry, you can easily determine if fire energy is filling your brain or if you have good water-fire energy circulation.

OPEN THE ENERGY BLOCKAGES IN THE HIPS

Sitting too much also leads to the brain overheating. Of course, it's different if you're sitting in meditation, circulating the energy in your body as you attune your breathing. Generally, however, sitting for a long time, staring at a computer, TV, or smartphone, is a fatally bad habit, one that inhibits water-fire circulation. In a seated posture, your hip joints fold, preventing the fire energy in the upper body from descending smoothly into the lower body. Respiration grows shallower and faster over time, continuously driving fire energy into the head.

You can easily test how sitting and standing affect your energy balance. First, sit in a chair or on a sofa for three to five minutes and observe your breathing and energy state. Is your breath growing deeper or more shallow as time passes? Is heat moving up into your head or down? If you concentrate on the place where your hips are folded, you'll recognize that the energy of your upper body isn't moving smoothly down into your lower body.

Now get up. Stand for three to five minutes, observing the state of your breathing and energy. Is your breathing growing deeper or more shallow with time? Is heat moving up into your head or down? Do you feel that the energy of your upper body moves down into your lower body better with your hip joints unfolded than when you were sitting down?

As we can see from this simple test, if you feel that your brain is overheated, you should get up immediately and move your body. You don't necessarily need to do hard exercise. It's also good to do simple household chores like cooking, dishwashing, and cleaning, things you can easily do as part of your daily life. Move your body that way for a while, and before you realize it, you'll discover that your thoughts have subsided and the heat in your head has naturally gone down into your lower body.

Walking is better than anything else for cooling the brain. Try going outdoors and walking for just 20 to 30 minutes. Walking makes the legs pass back and forth repeatedly, which exercises the hip joints and eliminates any energy bottlenecks there. The heat in the upper body sinks into the lower body more readily once any blockages in the hips are resolved.

When you walk, try focusing on breathing out. The heat in your head will leave your body along with your exhaled breath. And try to feel your breathing automatically sinking deep into your lower abdomen as your hip joints, hip muscles, and intestines are worked. If you check your head's temperature after walking, you'll find that it has cooled down. See page 112 for specific walking tips.

The following exercises will help you release tension from your hip joints. Especially if you have to sit for a lengthy time while working or reading, I recommend that you stand at least once every 30 minutes to open the energy blockages in your hips.

HIP JOINT TAPPING

In a standing posture, use your closed fists to tap your hip joints for about a minute, front and back. This is most effective if you exhale as you tap.

HIP JOINT STRETCHING

1. Stand with your hands on your hips and bend your upper body to one side, trying to feel your hip joint stretching.

2. Now do the same thing on the other side.

3. Stretch your upper body forward and backward as well several times.

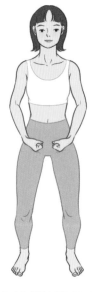

HIP JOINT TAPPING

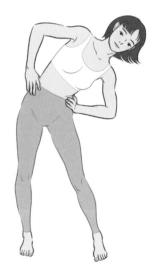

HIP JOINT STRETCHING

HIP JOINT ROTATIONS

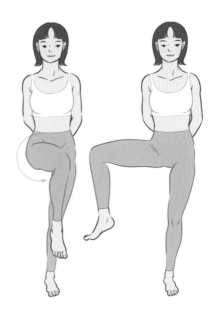

1. Stand and raise one leg, knee bent to hip height.

2. Use the hip on that side to make as big a circle as possible with your bent leg.

3. Do 10 circles clockwise and 10 counterclockwise.

4. Now switch sides and do the exercise with your other leg. If you have trouble maintaining your balance, you can place one hand on a wall for support.

After Exercising: Standing where you are with eyes closed, stabilize your breathing and try to detect what's happening in your body—the state of your energy. Do you feel the heat from the hip area spreading to your lower back, buttocks, and lower belly? Do you get the sense that your hip blockages have been reduced? Does it feel like the energy circulation in your upper and lower body is improving? Do you feel your breathing deepening and fire energy sinking?

RELEASE ENERGY STAGNATION IN YOUR HEAD

When heat rushes to the head, tension increases in the head and neck. Conversely, when tension increases in the head and neck, heat more readily rushes to the head. Accordingly, reducing tension in the head and neck helps heat in the head move downward.

A considerable number of energy points are located in the head and neck. Of the 14 major meridians, eight pass this spot: the Governing Vessel (Water Way), Conception Vessel (Fire Way), Bladder, Stomach, Gallbladder, Small Intestine, Large Intestine, and Triple Burner meridians.

The following exercises have the effect of opening energy blockages in the energy points and meridians of the head, speeding circulation of energy throughout the body. Once energy is unblocked and circulating, the heat that had flooded the head naturally sinks, moving down the body.

TAPPING ENERGY POINTS ON THE HEAD

Tap your head with your fingertips, as shown in the figure. It's critical to keep exhaling while tapping. Concentrate on your outgoing breath, imagining heat and stagnant energy leaving your head through your exhalations.

1. First, tap the crown of your head about 30 times; then move forward and down, tapping along the centerline of your head.

2. Now tap evenly around the top of your head. Then tap in sequence on the sides, back, and lower back of your head (where the head and neck meet). Concentrate your tapping on any points that feel especially painful.

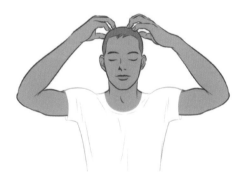

PRESSING ENERGY POINTS ON THE HEAD

Once you've discharged the heat from your head through tapping, you can move on to pressing your head's energy points. You can press with the tips of your fingers or with a tool—either the BHP Finder (Brain Education Healing Point Finder, designed especially for this) or the blunt end of a pen cap.

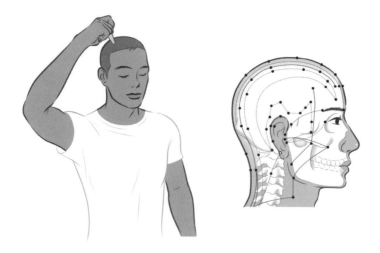

1. First stimulate the energy points all over your head by firmly pressing the top, sides, and back of your head with all your fingers.

2. Now press the same places using a tool or your fingernails. Refer to the chart of energy points above, but press most intensely on any areas where you feel pain, focusing on your bodily sensations.

3. If you discover places where pain is especially intense, those are the points that need healing. The pain results from severe energy stagnation in that point. Concentrate on relieving those spots to improve energy circulation.

After Exercising: With your eyes closed and your breathing relaxed and deep, try to detect what's happening in your body—the state of your energy. Does your head feel cooler and lighter than before? Does it feel like the heat in your head has lessened? Is your mouth filling with saliva, and are your eyes moister?

Pressing energy points on the head is first aid you can use as soon as you feel your head full of heat and pressure. After doing this for several minutes, you'll find yourself yawning and your eyes watering as the heat leaves your head.

RELAX THE TENSION IN YOUR NECK MUSCLES

When stressed, people typically hold the back of their necks. That's because this is the area that tenses up first. When that happens, the medulla oblongata in the lower back part of the skull, which controls respiration, is stimulated, resulting in shallower, faster breathing. And when breathing isn't smooth, energy circulation throughout the body is obstructed, resulting in reversed water-fire flow and pushing heat into the head. Since the neck is an important place along the Water Way, tension at the back of the neck also interferes with the rising of water energy.

Relaxing your neck muscles is a shortcut to stabilizing your breathing and restoring water-fire energy flow. If you want to ensure that you have good water-fire balance in your everyday life, it's important to pay attention to whether your neck muscles are tense. Try doing the following exercises whenever you feel your head growing hot and heavy.

NECK STRETCHING

1. Stretch the muscles on the left side of your neck while tilting your head to the right for 10 seconds.

2. Now do the same thing on the other side.

3. Next, interlocking your fingers behind your head, pull your head forward and down as far as you can. You'll feel the stretch in the muscles of your shoulders and back as well as the back of your neck.

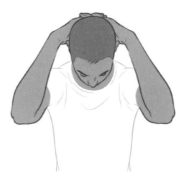

NECK ROTATIONS

1. Relax the tension in your neck by rotating it slowly three times in one direction.

2. Now do the same thing in the opposite direction.

3. Next, tilting your head back, move your neck to the left and right, relaxing tension in the muscles along the back of the neck and top of the shoulders.

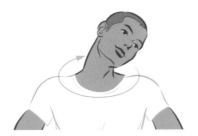

PRESSING ENERGY POINTS
AT THE BACK OF THE NECK

In sequence, use your thumbs to press or massage (in a circular motion) the energy points along the line where your head and neck meet (refer to the diagram for specific points). Imagine your breathing improving as the tension is released there, activating the functions of the medulla oblongata.

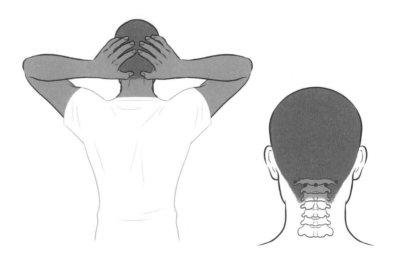

RELAXING MUSCLES AT THE BACK OF THE NECK

1. Bring one hand to the back of your neck, as shown in the figure below.

2. Relax the muscles right beside your cervical vertebrae by massaging them with your fingers. Taking your time, carefully relax all the tension in the muscles at the back of your neck, top to bottom.

3. Switching your hands, now do the other side.

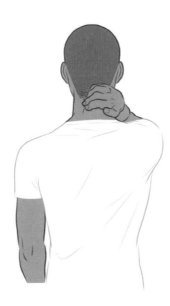

After Exercising: After doing these four exercises, close your eyes to discern the condition and energy state of your body. Does it feel like more heat has gone down from your head, neck, and face? Is your neck more relaxed, your breathing deeper and more stable?

If you deepen your breathing for a while after you've released the energy stagnation in your head and neck, you will be able to experience the water energy rising from your kidneys to slowly cool your head. The saliva gradually filling your mouth is a sign that you are recovering Water Up, Fire Down energy circulation.

CHAPTER 11
Develop the Power of Your Mind

I've stressed it repeatedly, but I'll say it again. The state of your mind determines the state of your energy.

The state of your mind determines the depth and quality of your breathing, and your breathing circulates your energy. Anxiety causes rapid, shallow breathing, inhibiting energy circulation, while peace of mind promotes slow, deep breathing, bringing energy circulation and balance to your whole body. Your energy circulation and balance determine your physical health, your breathing determines the state of your energy, and your mind determines the quality of your breathing. It is no exaggeration to say that your mind is the key to maintaining your water-fire energy balance and your health.

What can you do to maintain peace of mind, then? I suggest that you develop your "heart power"—the power of your mind to remain unshaken in all circumstances.

Yes, heart power is something you can have, a hidden superpower, you might say. Heart power isn't something you can gain just by making up your mind to do so, however. Overly firm resolve often leads to stubbornness, self-righteousness, or a tight grip on how you think things should be. To develop heart power, you need to find your heart's true center. But what is the heart's true center? It is who you are in the most basic sense, your true self. To have heart power, you have to find out what that is and make that the center of your mind.

Finding and building your heart power starts with a simple question: "Who am I?" This is a very important question to ask, and as long as you do so sincerely, it can help you get to the essence of your being. To get the answer to this question, you have to go beyond the things listed on your driver's license and the details decorating your resume. Your true self is your true nature—your pure, unaltered character—not something you've gained or achieved. It's the part of you that was already with you when you were a tiny child and that will be there on your last day on earth. If you can sense this part of your being, then you are on your way to finding your heart power.

Your true self is the unadulterated, true nature dwelling within you like clear, deep, blue water, unchanging from moment to moment, unaffected by anyone or anything. The world and your emotions are like a storm that causes the waves on the surface to become rough, but your true self is like the calm waters far below. Having the heart power that comes from your true self is like having a strong keel on your boat that allows you to keep upright even in the worst conditions.

When we say we suffer because of something or someone, it's generally because we've switched focus from our primary identity, our true self, toward some secondary identity. If this happens, our priorities switch from concerns of the true self to concerns of the outside world. With the mind taken over by secondary priorities, our true center is inevitably veiled, and it loses its power.

Of course, I'm not telling you that secondary things are not important or that you shouldn't concern yourself with them at all. But it's enough to treat secondary things as, well, secondary. After first centering yourself solidly in your true nature, just treat everything else as something to be used, tools for your journey through life. Don't let your center be diminished, overwhelmed by the power of secondary things.

The stresses that undermine people's health often come from solely focusing on secondary priorities. Without a solid connection with their true selves, many chase what people think of them, how to get the material things they want, or when they will get the recognition they desire. I'm not talking about people whose basic needs for food and shelter have not been satisfied. Most people in our society are stressed out even though they have plenty to eat and warm beds to sleep in every night.

Always remember that the only thing you can take with you when you leave this world is your true nature. Genuine satisfaction can only come when you develop the energy of your true nature and make that the primary value of your life. No one has ever felt lasting satisfaction through only secondary things like fame and money, so never drop your primary value for grasping less important things in your life.

You might think of the information or influences that weaken the connection to your true nature as harmful energies that invade your mind. Just like your body has an immune system, you need to develop the immunity of your mind. The body's immunity is its ability to maintain homeostasis by blocking the invasion of hazardous microorganisms such as bacteria and viruses. Similarly, your mental immunity maintains your peace of mind by protecting you from unhelpful information, keeping you focused on your most deeply held values. Your mental immune system is your ability to achieve equanimity, a mind that's not easily shaken in any situation.

Where do you usually have your mind centered? If there's something you're especially focused on, that is your mind's center. If you are experiencing constant stress or imbalance and can't find a way out of them, your mind may be too occupied by secondary things; for example, growing desires for material success, fame, relationships, or negative thoughts and emotions. Those things continuously eat up our attention, time, and energy, so you have to learn to let them go and let them occupy a secondary position in your life. This doesn't mean you have to keep low goals or kill your dreams. It does mean that establishing the center of your mind around your true self will save you from unnecessary suffering.

Greed is the endless desire to get more and more things in life, whether they are material, emotional, or mental. We have a basic drive to want things that we don't have. But if we are not mindful about it, it can become a deadly power, pulling us away from our center. It's simply impossible to satisfy greed because it just keeps wanting more. Greed produces attachment to the things and people we want to keep. If we constantly feed our greed and attachment, they will end up sitting in the front seat of our lives.

The world tells us that more money, new relationships, or a stack of knowledge will make us feel happy and secure, but we know that they don't last. Soon we become anxious again to go after the next big exciting thing.

Those who have discovered their true selves and have made that the firm center of their minds are undisturbed by changes in their external environment or by the effects of negative information. They are able to maintain peace of mind because of the powerful actions of their mental immunity. Check yourself: "Am I centered in my true nature, or is my desire for secondary things dragging me away from it?"

You will be able to center your mind when you let go of the desires you once clung to so tightly. Peace of mind can only come to dwell in an empty state of mind, a place free of ever-growing greed and its mental representations. Hoping to have peace of mind when your mind is full of all sorts of complicated desires is impossible, so do your best to re-center and let go of your grip on the things that disconnect you from your true self.

When you are aware of a greedy feeling or an attachment that makes you anxious, stop and ask yourself, "Do I really need this? Is this what my true self wants?" Let go of your excessive greed for anything that does not serve your true center—status, success, leisure, food—anything that distances you from your genuine self. Then, start developing the energy of your true nature and make it the center of your mind. Only then can your mind be truly powerful and maintain your well-being through water-fire energy balance.

The three meditation practices that follow are meant to help you develop your heart power and protect the energy of your true nature. It's good to do these in succession. But first, check the power of your mind.

Before You Begin: Check the Power of Your Mind

1. Do you tend to be swayed by changes in your environment or by external information?

How do you respond when you're faced with some change or confronted by negative information? Do you feel bad or become anxious, easily influenced by these things? Or do you have the mental power to watch such changes dispassionately?

2. Does your negative consciousness tend to be strong?

Although negative consciousness does develop when negative information comes in from the outside, it is also created internally. When you are facing a difficult situation and are uncertain about your future, do you tend to keep expanding your thoughts and feelings in a negative direction? Or do you have the mental strength to comfort yourself, letting go of negative information and switching to a positive, proactive state of mind?

3. Do you have faith in yourself, and is your mind centered?

Do you have faith in yourself, or do you tend to be anxious and worried, unable to trust yourself? Do you usually trust and tolerate other people well, or are you on your guard, unable to trust others? Do you have your own values and a belief system that keeps you centered and unshaken when faced with difficult circumstances?

LAY DOWN YOUR ATTACHMENTS

1. Sit in a chair or in a meditation posture on the floor. Straighten your lower back, place your hands on your knees, palms up, and then close your eyes.

2. Look into your heart and sense the feeling there. Do you feel endless comfort and peace or a tangled, painful mess?

3. Look more closely. Are you clinging to ideas, memories, or emotions that make you suffer, or are you able to handle them wisely? If they cause you to suffer and you no longer want them to, then it's time to let them go.

4. Breathe in through your nose and then exhale through your mouth, "Hoo ....." Imagine fresh air and energy entering and filling your chest when you breathe in and the energy of emotions, attachments, and greed leaving your heart when you breathe out.

5. With each breath, visualize your heart gradually being emptied of the energies of attachment and greed that have been knotted up inside. As heavy energy leaves, your chest slowly opens, becoming lighter. Continue until your chest feels sufficiently light and unburdened.

DEVELOP THE ENERGY OF YOUR TRUE SELF

1. Sit in a chair or on the floor in a half-lotus position. Raise your hands in front of your chest to send energy into your heart as you did in Chapter 9 to send healing energy to your chest (page 133).

2. Imagine your palms emitting pure energy and transmitting it into your chest. Your true self is there. Send energy to your true nature, your true center. The energy is bound to go where you send it. Continue to develop the energy of your true nature.

3. Keep sending energy into your chest until your heart feels full of the energy of your true nature.

4. As you imagine a vortex of energy forming in the middle of your chest, try talking with the energy of your true nature: "Oh, my true nature, I'll now make you the solid center of my being. I won't let go of you, no matter what situation comes. I now understand that it is you who can give me true peace and satisfaction. Please always protect me there in my heart. Will you be my strong friend and companion? I'm delighted and overjoyed to have you. Thank you, energy of my true nature."

PROTECT YOURSELF WITH AN ENERGY CAPSULE

1. Sitting in a chair or on the floor with your lower back straight and your eyes closed, bring your palms in front of your face. Leave about one inch of space between your palms and your face. Imagine energy coming out of your palms and going into your face; you may feel a pleasant sense of warmth in your face. As that is gradually amplified, energy is being activated in different parts of your face, which will wear an ever-widening smile.

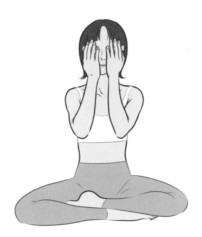

2. Within your body flows a bioelectromagnetic field commonly called an aura. The heat and energy you feel now is that electromagnetic field. Moving your hands in very, very slow circles, gradually amplify the energy field flowing between your face and hands. Imagine that field slowly expanding and intensifying.

3. If the flow of energy is blocked in your face area, try stretching your facial muscles as much as possible when sending energy there. Spread them to the sides—the muscles of your forehead, eyes, nose, mouth, cheeks, and chin—and open your mouth as wide as possible with an "Ah . . . ." As you do that, continue sending healing energy from your palms to your face. The darker your expression normally is, the more you'll be able to feel the once-contracted muscles of your face gradually relaxing and expanding.

4. Now heal the energy field of your head. Moving your hands very, very slowly, send energy into the area around your head—as if you are putting on a helmet made of energy. Stretch the muscles of your head, making a really big smile. Send energy evenly to the front, sides, top, and back of your head. Your head's energy field is slowly healing and being amplified.

5. Next, use one hand to send energy to the area around the opposite arm. Amplify the energy of that arm as if you're wearing an energy glove. Now switch hands and do the same thing for your other arm.

6. Move on to your chest and trunk. Strengthen your energy field by moving your hands very slowly down from your chest to your lower abdomen. Focus on sending energy anywhere that feels like it needs healing or where your energy field feels weak, circling your palms very slowly over those spots.

7. Extend your legs and slowly move your hands from your abdomen to your toes, intensifying your energy field. Heal and stroke every nook and cranny of your energy field, including the sides and backs of your legs.

8. Now slowly sit in a meditation posture. Hold your hands, palms up, about five inches above your knees. Leave space between your arms and sides, and also leave space between your fingers.

9. With your eyes closed, straighten your lower back. Imagine and try to feel the bioelectromagnetic field surrounding your body growing stronger. Try to visualize the energy field around your body being activated in a round globe, as if you're an energy snowman. An energy capsule surrounds your body.

10. Now focus your mind on the crown of your head. Imagine the energy of the universe—cosmic energy—pouring down into the top of your head. Visualize it coming down, passing through your chest, descending into your lower abdomen, and flowing our of your body in a single line.

11. Cosmic energy flows from your head into the palms of your hands. Focus your mind on your palms, feeling hot energy there, too. Then feel three energy pillars forming, one into your head and one into each palm. Continue being charged with cosmic energy.

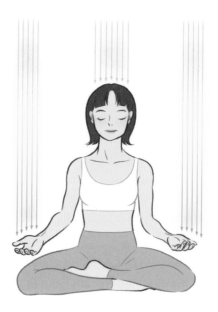

12. Focus your mind on your lower dahnjon. Imagine it being charged by hot cosmic energy. In your mind, silently call out "dahnjon" three times as energy slowly fills your dahnjon, heating it. Visualize cosmic energy continuing to descend, heating your dahnjon, fanning its flames.

13. Imagine the energy of the lower dahnjon in your belly shining with a red light, the energy of your middle dahnjon in your chest shining with a golden light, and the energy of

your upper dahnjon in your head shining with a blue light. Visualize these three energy centers charged with cosmic energy, now activated and emitting a bright light. Your energy capsule, charged and perfect, will protect you.

After Exercising: Maintaining your meditation posture, feel the state of energy in your body. Does your belly feel warmer, your chest more comfortable, and your head cooler than before? Does your breathing feel more comfortable, deeper, and more stable? Does the energy axis from the top of your head to your perineum feel strong, and does your mind feel more powerful?

I suggest that you do this Energy Capsule Meditation once a day. We eat every day, supplementing our bodies with nutrients and calories, but that is not enough. To strengthen the central axis of our minds and our three energy centers, we need time every day to recharge with the fundamental life energy of the universe. Then, our deep hunger, somehow unsatisfied by even three meals a day, will finally be satiated. Our limited energy is discharged as we use it, but we can recharge with the infinite energy of the cosmos whenever we need to.

I want to share with you the Cosmic Energy Message in which I expressed the feelings I had when my whole body was charged with cosmic energy. If you think of this when you're filled up with cosmic energy during Energy Capsule Meditation, its effects will be amplified further. Remember once again this great principle: Where your mind goes, energy follows.

Cosmic Energy Message

Cosmic energy brings health of body and peace of mind.

Cosmic energy eliminates loneliness and sadness.

Cosmic energy brings calm and confidence.

Cosmic energy fills your empty mind with love.

*Cosmic energy gives you the strength to forgive
even those who've caused you pain.*

With cosmic energy, there is no fear.

With cosmic energy, there is no dread.

*Within cosmic energy, there is no victim
consciousness, selfishness, or conceit.*

*Cosmic energy changes us into diligent,
responsible, honest people.*

*Cosmic energy is the sacred breath of the universe
that clears the spirit and develops the soul,
bringing spiritual completion.*

CHAPTER 12

Establish Your Own Water Up, Fire Down Routine

S o far, I've introduced specific methods you can use to resolve three conditions hindering water-fire energy circulation: stress-related overheating of the head, energy stagnation in the chest, and weakness of the core. And I've presented methods of meditation for developing the power of your mind, your ultimate tool for energy balance. Now, it's time to build your own water-fire energy routine based on the principles and methods in this book.

All the training methods I've suggested are effective and powerful, but it's not easy to do all of them every day. Why don't you build your own daily water-fire energy routine by choosing several that are effective for you and fit your situation and condition?

The 24-hour day is the most important unit of time in our lives. We set goals based on different units—week, month, year, decade— but none of these is as important as a single day for taking substantial action. This applies to health as well. The basis of good health is how you live a single day. If you neglect something one day, before you know it, several more days have passed, making it harder to recover disrupted habits and life rhythms.

Creating a healthy day is possible for everyone. If you thought you had to be healthy and free of sickness your whole life, it might seem an insurmountable task, but spending one day—today— following good health practices is doable. Those days accumulate, becoming your entire life. Practice water-fire circulation today for your health right now. The surest way to apply to your life the Golden Principle of Health—Water Up, Fire Down energy circula- tion—is to create a routine and repeat it daily.

When you create your water-fire circulation routine, incorpo- rate these three elements sequentially:

Step 1. Open your energy blockages.

Step 2. Warm your lower belly.

Step 3. Control your breathing.

Think of it this way. If boiler pipes are blocked, preventing circu- lation, it's best to eliminate the blockage before turning on the pump. The same principle applies to our bodies. Start by using methods to release blockages in the back of your neck, chest, and Joongwan—places where energy is easily blocked. If you have the time, it's best to do your training for releasing blockages after first stretching to relax all the muscles and joints of your body.

After you break through blockages, then warm your lower belly. Raising the temperature of your abdomen improves the functioning of all your organs, enhances your immune function, and produces a natural circulation of energy in your body. It also naturally cools down your overheated head. Dahnjon Tapping, Intestinal Exercise, and Belly Button Healing are good examples of exercises for warming your belly. They are also good for opening your blockages and releasing tension.

Find some time to breathe after giving enough warmth to your belly. With your breathing deep and stable, observe the vital phenomena arising in your body. Then your mind will settle as your thoughts and emotions naturally subside. Use the meditation methods in this book to deepen your breathing. Energy Capsule Meditation in particular will help you find peace of mind and stabilize your breathing.

Release blockages in your neck, chest, and Joongwan to open your energy pipeline. Move your belly to activate your lower body's energy heat pump. And control your breathing to circulate energy efficiently to your entire body. Then water-fire energy flow will develop naturally, creating an optimal life-enhancing environment in which your brain and body can function well. If you apply these basic principles in the correct sequence, even when you've developed reversed water-fire flow due to stress, you'll be able to rapidly recover a normal condition.

On the following pages, I've presented a training flow appropriate for mornings and evenings as an example of a water-fire energy workout routine. You could also come up with your own creative routines by using some of the exercises in this book or combining them with health routines you're already doing.

The water-fire energy exercises you do in the morning will help you have a great day, full of vitality. A day started by taking time to interact with your body is quite different from one begun in a rush, huffing and puffing as if you're being pursued. It would be good if you could take about 20 to 30 minutes early in the day to do a morning routine. If you're too busy for that in the morning, make sure you set aside at least 20 to 30 minutes in the evening. Do you remember the strategy for managing stress that I talked about in Chapter 5? Don't take the day's stress to bed with you.

It's important to take the time to purify your energy before you go to bed. Going to sleep in a stressed state is particularly bad. If the energy of negative emotions builds up and isn't released, your Fire Way will remain blocked, and it will take a long time to purify your energy. I'm in the habit of saying, half-jokingly, that you should take time to cleanse your energy before going to bed, even if you don't shower. That's how crucial energy management is. You need a shower to wash away the day's fatigue and stress, not just to cleanse your body. The water-fire energy evening routine introduced in these pages will help you release the fatigue built up during the day and go to sleep with a comfortable body and mind, your energy balanced.

MORNING ROUTINE

The following morning routine promotes physical vitality through exercises to circulate and activate the stagnated energy of a body that has been lying down all night. Afterward, I recommend doing the Energy Capsule Meditation in Chapter 11 for preparing the body and mind to start the day.

Step 1-1. Joint Rotations

You can release energy blockages by rotating the joints where energy points are concentrated and energy stagnation readily occurs. The aim is to slowly circle your joints, making the circles as large as possible, while getting a feel for the condition of your body, including your joints and surrounding muscles. I've given a suggested number of repetitions for each joint, but you don't need to feel bound by that—adjust the exercise to your own condition. You can do the neck, shoulder, and wrist rotations sitting down if you would like.

NECK ROTATIONS

Rotate your neck three times slowly in one direction and then in the other. Stretch your neck and bend your head as far back as you can. Then move it from side to side, relaxing the tension in the back of your neck.

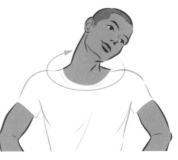

SHOULDER ROTATIONS

Rotate your shoulders, lifting them up as far as possible and then moving them back, down, forward, and upward again. Do five rotations from front to back, then reverse the direction of your movement and do five from back to front. Make your circles as large as you can in order to stimulate both the muscles and the joints of your shoulders, neck, chest, and back.

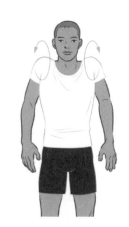

WRIST ROTATIONS

Stretching your arms out in front of your body, slowly rotate your wrists. Turn them 10 times in one direction and then 10 times in the other direction.

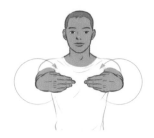

HIP ROTATIONS

Place your hands on your hips, and then bend your upper body forward and rotate your hips, moving them in as large a circle as possible. As you do the hip rotations, feel your hip joints and the muscles of your buttocks, lower back, and legs being stimulated and stretched. Do five repetitions in each direction.

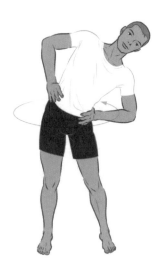

KNEE ROTATIONS

With your hands on your knees, move them together in circles for five times in each direction. Then let your knees separate and move them in circles, five times from the inside out and then five times from the outside in.

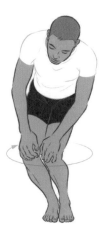

ANKLE ROTATIONS

Raising one heel and keeping your knees loose, slowly rotate the ankle of that foot five times in one direction. Repeat in the other direction. Now do the same thing with the other foot.

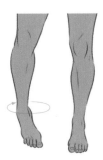

Step 1-2. Stretching

This exercise includes basic movements that stretch the front, sides, and back of the body to open energy blockages.

SIDE STRETCHING

Stretching sideways stimulates the Gallbladder Meridian that flows along the sides of the body.

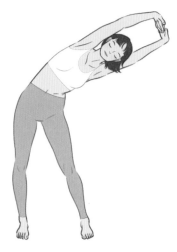

1. Clasp your hands and raise them above your head as far as you can.

2. Then bend your torso to one side.

3. Hold that posture for about five seconds, feeling the stretch.

4. Now bend toward the other side and hold for five seconds.

CHEST AND BACK STRETCHING

Blockages of the Fire Way in the chest and the Water Way in the back are released by this movement.

1. Stand balanced with your feet shoulder-width apart and your knees slightly bent.

2. Place your clasped hands behind your head and bend your head and shoulders backward.

3. Moving your elbows back as much as possible, press forward with your chest.

4. Now do the opposite, bending your head, arms, and upper body as far forward as you can. Feel the muscles in the back of your neck, spine, and back being stretched.

5. Alternating these movements, do three repetitions of each.

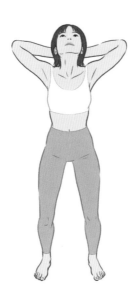

HAMSTRING STRETCH

This stretch effectively stimulates the Bladder Meridian that flows along the back of the body.

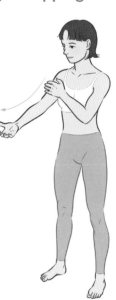

1. With your feet together, let your buttocks move backward as you push your clasped hands forward as far as you can.

2. Hold that posture for 10 seconds, feeling the stretch at the back of your legs.

3. Continue to push your hands outward, slowly lowering them toward your feet. Hold that posture, with your hands pushing down as far as possible, and feel the Bladder Meridian at the back of your legs being stretched.

Step 2. Full-Body Tapping and Dahnjon Tapping

FULL-BODY TAPPING

This exercise, which involves tapping every part of your body along your meridians, stimulates all 12 meridians and awakens the cells of your body.

1. Standing with your left arm raised, palm facing up, use your right hand to tap your left arm from shoulder to palm (Heart and Pericardium Meridians).

2. Now turn your left palm down and tap the outside of your left arm from the back of the hand to the shoulder (Triple Burner Meridian).

3. Turning your left thumb upward, tap your arm from shoulder to thumb (Large Intestine and Lung Meridians), then from little finger to armpit (Small Intestine Meridian).

4. Tap your other arm in the same sequence.

5. Tap your chest with both hands to open your Fire Way, and then tap your stomach on your left side and your liver on your right side (Stomach and Liver Meridians).

6. Bending forward, tap your kidneys and buttocks, and then tap down along the back of your legs (Bladder Meridian).

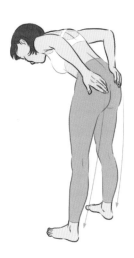

7. Starting with your feet, tap up along the front of both legs (Stomach and Spleen Meridians).

8. Starting at your hips, tap down along the outside of both legs (Gallbladder Meridian).

9. Starting at your ankles, tap up along the inside of both legs (Liver and Kidney Meridians).

DAHNJON TAPPING

After doing full-body tapping, go immediately into Dahnjon Tapping. Standing, bend your knees slightly and pat your lower dahnjon with the palms of your hands. Strike forcefully enough to make a drumming sound. Do about 100 repetitions.

If your situation dictates that you shouldn't make noise while doing Dahnjon Tapping, do the exercise using alternating fists (see page 105), or do Intestinal Exercise and Belly Button Healing instead (see page 107).

Step 3. Energy Capsule Meditation

Sitting in a meditation posture, do abdominal breathing. As your abdomen expands and contracts on its own, feel your breath coming deep into your gut. Feel the cells of your whole body awaken and the energy of your body be activated.

In this state, do Energy Capsule Meditation (see page 161). First, send energy to your face using the palms of your hands. Stretch your facial muscles as much as possible to start your day with a bright smile. Imagine your energy field growing more robust as you send energy to your head and every part of your body. Visualizing yourself surrounded by a capsule of energy, charge and circulate its bright, powerful energy. Through this process, your body, mind, and energy will be readied to start the day. Don't forget to send yourself a positive, hopeful message, one of gratitude for the day you've been given.

EVENING ROUTINE

In the evening, if you do stretching to release the day's fatigue and tension, Joongwan Healing and Belly Button Healing to induce deep breathing, and then Energy Capsule Meditation, you'll be perfectly prepared to go to bed wrapped in a blanket of refreshed energy.

Step 1. Stretching

Since you'll be tired in the evening, this routine uses exercises effective for relaxing the tension built up during the day, centered on stretches done in a lying position.

LEG CROSSOVERS

1. Lie on your back with your arms at your sides stretched higher than your shoulders.

2. Raise your left leg, knee bent, and cross it over your body to the right. Use your right hand to press your knee down.

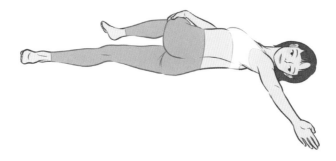

3. Hold this posture for one to two minutes, feeling the stretch in your side, lower back, chest, shoulders, armpit, and arm. Relaxing as you continue exhaling, you may find yourself yawning as exhausted energy is discharged from your brain.

4. Do the same thing on the other side.

5. You may experience numbness in your arms as stagnant energy is released from places that have been tense and blocked. If this happens, switch to working the other side.

KNEE PULL-INS

1. Lying on your back, bend your knees and clasp your hands over them.

2. Alternately pull your knees to your chest and let them bounce back. Do this 20 times.

3. Now inhale, again pulling in your bent legs. Bring them as close as you can to your chest while lifting your head to your knees at the same time. Hold this position for five seconds, feeling your back stretching.

4. Release as you exhale. Repeat three to five times.

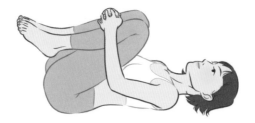

PLOW POSE

1. From a lying position, lift your legs back over your head and hold your feet with your hands. If this is too difficult, place your hands against your lower back for support as you keep your legs raised.

2. Emphasize your exhale, feeling your shoulders and back being stretched. Hold this position for a minute if you can.

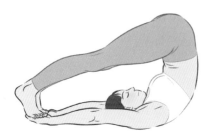

KNEELING SHOULDER STRETCH

1. Kneel with your ankles flexed and toes on the ground. Bend your upper body forward, placing the palms of your hands on the floor.

2. Pressing forward with your hands, lower your chest as far as you can and touch your chin to the floor.

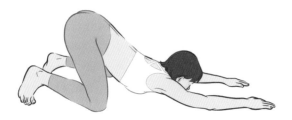

3. Hold this position for one to two minutes, feeling the stretch in your shoulders, chest, and thoracic vertebrae.

COBRA POSE

1. Lying face down on the floor with your hands under your shoulders and your toes pointed, slowly extend your arms to raise your upper body, then tilt your head back.

2. Hold this position for one to two minutes, feeling the stretch in your neck, chest, hips, and lower back.

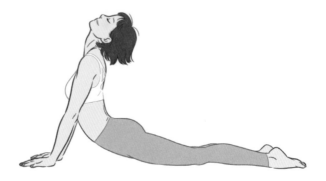

Step 2. Joongwan Healing and Belly Button Healing

In a seated posture, pump your Joongwan point about 100 times using your hands or a tool, as described on page 126. Continue pressing deeply as you exhale, hold for about five seconds, and then relax and hold your breath for another five seconds. Repeat 5 to 10 times. Your third chakra, which tensed during the day, will relax. Next, pump your belly button about 100 times. You can easily make your breathing descend into your abdomen as your intestines become more pliable. As you relax your attention into your respiration, do deep abdominal breathing.

Step 3. Energy Capsule Meditation

Once your breathing has become deeper, you can continue on to Energy Capsule Meditation. See page 161 for detailed instructions.

Deeply stretch your facial muscles as you transmit energy into your face with your hands, sending yourself bright, positive energy. Concentrate on sending healing energy into any fatigued organs or painful areas of your body, imagining yourself repairing your energy field in those places. Comfort and encourage yourself after a day's hard work as you evenly massage the energy field of your whole body, and imagine it changing gradually into a full, complete capsule. You'll be comfortable and ready for a good night's sleep, your energy cleansed and refreshed.

FUNDAMENTAL MEDITATIONS

If you have trouble feeling the subtle currents of energy in your body, I'm including a method that lets you sense energy directly. Since the principle of Water Up, Fire Down concerns the flow and circulation of energy, you can achieve energy balance much more effectively if you know ways to feel and control energy. I've briefly introduced a method of abdominal breathing as well. As you do your water-fire energy routine every day, your breathing will gradually deepen and sink into your belly. The abdominal breathing method presented here will foster your water-fire energy balance.

FEELING ENERGY

To feel energy directly, start by feeling the energy in your hands, the most sensitive place in your body. Your energy sense will develop gradually, and once that happens, you can feel energy spreading into your arms, your chest, and your whole body.

In order to do this, you need to focus on very subtle energy sensations, with your body and mind as relaxed as possible and your brain waves stable. As a preparatory step, do some light stretching followed by Dahnjon Tapping, Joongwan Healing, or Belly Button Healing to ensure that your energy sinks down into your abdomen, stabilizing and deepening your breathing.

1. Sit in a chair or on the floor in a half-lotus or other comfortable meditation posture. Straighten your lower back and place your hands on your knees, palms up. Close your eyes and breathe comfortably.

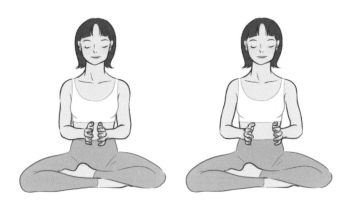

2. When your breathing is stable, slowly bring your hands in front of your chest. Touch your fingertips to each other and tap them together about 50 times.

3. Next, rub your palms together rapidly for about 10 to 20 seconds, generating heat there.

4. Then stop and move your palms apart so they are facing each other with about one inch between them.

5. Gently close your eyes and focus on the feelings in your hands. They may feel hot, your fingertips may tingle, or it may feel like something is crawling between your fingers. Those are sensations of energy.

6. Repeatedly move your palms slightly apart and then back together. Let yourself be immersed in the sensations in

your hands, very slowly and repeatedly expanding and contracting the space between them. Those who are very sensitive to energy will sense heat and magnetism between their hands being amplified, like they have an air balloon between their palms or their hands are pulling and pushing against each other.

7. Now move your hands slightly off-center, trying to roll the air balloon you seem to have between them. Think of the balloon as a ball of energy and try to turn it around, very slowly, between the palms of your hands. Imagine the energy ball growing larger and stronger as you focus on the feelings between your hands.

The first time you do this exercise, you may feel no sensations at all, or the feeling may be extremely slight. There could be many reasons for this, including your body and mind not being relaxed enough. Your ability to concentrate on your internal sensations may also still be weak, or your mind may lack focus, bombarded by too many distracting thoughts. Nevertheless, keep trying. If you practice activating and circulating your energy—doing the exercises introduced in the previous sections for strengthening your core, opening your chest, and lowering the heat in your head—your body and mind will relax more and more. Your concentration on your physical sensations will eventually improve, along with your ability to sense energy.

Don't expect to feel some incredible energy phenomena at the very beginning. Instead, look for small, subtle sensations, and allow them to expand and intensify as you practice. And remember, this is not a special talent granted only to some people. Anyone with an active brain sense can feel energy because our bodies themselves are made of energy. The differences among people are merely how developed their individual energy senses are. Just as we enhance the strength and flexibility of our bodies, we develop our energy sense through constant practice and concentration.

ABDOMINAL BREATHING

As I've mentioned previously, the best breathing for water-fire balance is abdominal breathing—inhaling and exhaling with your lower belly slowly and deeply. However, I don't recommend abdominal breathing for newcomers to water-fire energy training who haven't yet acquired a sense for feeling their bodies. Most people have a blocked Fire Way and stiff intestines, and they can easily get a stifling feeling in their chest or a headache if they try to do abdominal breathing in that condition. It's better to do it after first opening the Fire Way sufficiently by using Joongwan Healing and different methods for removing energy blockages in the chest, focusing on practices such as Intestinal Exercise and Dahnjon Tapping to relax the gut and warm the belly.

1. Sit on the floor or in a chair in a comfortable position and straighten your lower back. You can also lie on your back on a flat surface. Relax your neck, shoulders, and arms and close your eyes.

2. Place one hand on your chest and the other hand on your lower abdomen.

3. When you breathe in, let your abdomen expand like a balloon filling with air. When you exhale, let your abdomen contract. The hand on your chest should remain relatively still.

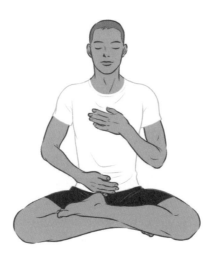

4. For beginners, it's good to start with focusing on the feeling of slowly pulling the abdomen in and out without worrying about the length of each breath.

5. Relax any tension in your body and mind, and breathe comfortably. You don't need to intentionally breathe slowly or hold your breath. Once your body is sufficiently relaxed, your breathing will automatically slow and stabilize.

6. As you continue doing abdominal breathing, you'll develop heat in your belly. Focus your mind on that heat, and it will gradually grow stronger, spreading to your entire abdomen and lower back. Your belly will also feel full of energy.

7. Once you're familiar with breathing this way, lower your hands and place them comfortably on your knees or at your side. Breathe only through your nose, if possible.

8. It's good to do abdominal breathing for three to five minutes one to three times a day if you're a beginner. Once you're comfortable with abdominal breathing, increase the time you spend doing it in your everyday life—when you're walking, working, driving, and resting, for instance.

Tip: If your breathing is difficult, labored, or painful, then something is wrong. The best breathing practice is the one that makes you comfortable in both body and mind. If you keep doing the different methods for generating water-fire energy circulation presented in this book, you'll find that your breathing will gradually sink from your chest into your lower abdomen. To do abdominal breathing effectively, practice Joongwan Healing often for opening your Fire Way and Intestinal Exercise for developing the strength and flexibility of your abdominal muscles and gut.

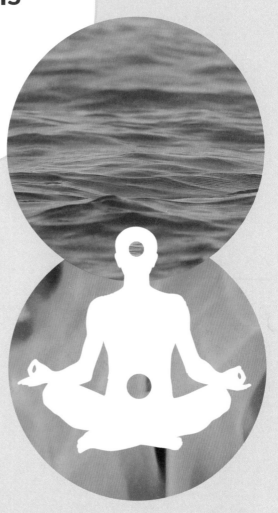

PART 3
Reflections

CHAPTER 13

Beyond Individual Energy Balance

This spring I have been staying at Earth Village in Kerikeri, New Zealand. Earth Village is where I am preparing to set up a residential school, a place where people can experience self-reliance and an environmentally friendly lifestyle. With all New Zealand in pandemic lockdown, I've also been sheltering in place. I love solitude and need time alone, but when people suddenly stopped coming to Earth Village, I really missed them. My heart was heavy with concern over how long the pandemic would last, where and how far the anxiety and fear sweeping the globe would drive us, and how the pandemic would change our lives and the earth. To find comfort, I have turned to a familiar friend—nature.

As I walk the woodland paths of Earth Village drinking in the fresh morning air and sit in a ravine listening to the flowing water and the sounds of my own breathing, my body achieves water-fire energy balance, and my mind's eye clears and expands. Even amid dramatic change, I feel the life force that brings balance and harmony to all things filling me, filling the universe. I feel that this power has never left us, even for an instant.

The great life force of nature is not with us only in the moments when we're overflowing with vigor and vitality. Even when unstoppable chaos sweeps the world, even when we are panicking, even when our lives hang in the balance, that power is with us. Our health and the well-being of the community can be restored when we vividly feel that power flowing through our bodies and connecting all things in creation.

When We Feel the Life Within

When we sit quietly with our eyes closed, controlling our breathing, the vital phenomenon of water-fire energy circulation grows vigorous in our bodies, and nature awakens within us. The ever-existing, uncreated, untamed essence of our true nature appears—not the personal brands we've been cultivating as we've lived our lives. We open our eyes to the value and preciousness of the life that has always existed in our bodies, and we become aware of who we are as we are, unadorned, regardless of all the artificial constructs we've made since being born into the world. Our occupations, money, personal relationships, success—things like these, although precious to us, lose their importance, subject to the vicissitudes of expanding and contracting values.

Trees in an exquisitely manicured garden are beautiful, but we find a unique beauty in trees that are growing wild in a field. Such trees comfort us for they are not artificial. Just as each tree shines with one-of-a-kind beauty, when the nature within us revives, we feel a "self" come alive as a unique, distinctive being—different from any other organism in this vast world. The joy of life, a joy that comes from existence itself, fills my heart as that happens. I feel that life has been given to me without condition, and I am truly grateful for it. Although I live as a being separate and independent from others, I feel with my whole body that I'm connected with all things through life. Welling up from that ardent sense of life is a longing for the well-being and peace of all people.

The joy, fullness, and gratitude that come to us when we vividly sense the life flowing within us—the absolute love for ourselves, unconditional and without reason—has tremendous healing power. The deep sense of connection with all beings given to us by the feeling of life grants us the strength to sincerely forgive and love ourselves and others. It melts away the disappointments and hurts we've experienced and lets us transcend any conflict, pain, and attachment coming from our relationships.

When the life within us awakens, we can truly own our lives, and we can create health and happiness for ourselves. We all have a sense of harmony and balance, a gift from nature. When we realize our water-fire energy balance is broken, we strive to restore it because we have this innate sense in our brains and bodies. That sense tells us what we need, what we should do now if we listen to our bodies and minds. It leads us to make choices that are good for the whole as well as for ourselves.

Secure Time for Balancing Your Energy Daily

Immersed in our busy daily lives, we easily forget the nature within us and remember only our feelings, thoughts, habits, and stories. We may work hard all day, busy producing many things, but we don't get inner satisfaction unless we feel our life force. We forget the joy that comes from life itself and seek to fill our emptiness with other people or material things. But as you know, it's hard to endure a life bereft of inner joy and satisfaction. The more joyless days we have, the more life feels like an endurance race, like we are killing time rather than living. When our minds remain too long in this condition, our bodies' energy flow flips, and we have reversed water-fire circulation.

That's why we must make time to connect with our essence in our daily lives. We need time to meet with nature, with the life force within us. The nature within us has always existed, and that's why it can never be destroyed. Our inner connection with nature may be momentarily broken, but that link cannot disappear. All we need to do is make up our minds to recover the connection.

All the methods of training for Water Up, Fire Down energy circulation introduced in this book are about taking the time to connect with nature inside you, with the life within, with your true nature. You can recover that connection even by quietly sensing the breath entering and leaving your body, by moving your body vigorously, feeling the rhythms of your heartbeat and the pleasant stiffness of your muscles, by focusing on your vital phenomena in this way.

I hope you will be able to create your own health and happiness by experiencing more Water Up, Fire Down energy flow, the astounding phenomenon of life inside you.

The Earth Needs Energy Balance, Too

Water Up, Fire Down energy circulation is necessary within ecosystems, just as it is necessary within the human body. Just as we experience physical sickness and emotional discomfort when we have reversed water-fire flow, nature suffers when its circulation is disrupted and its balance broken, for nature is a living organism, too. Our bodies have a natural healing ability for restoring our balance and harmony, but we can't avoid disease if we live in ways that suppress this power. Nature also has a fantastic capacity for purifying itself. Still, we keep injuring nature in profound ways, giving it no respite, no chance to heal the injuries we have inflicted upon it. The earth, like many people, is suffering burnout because of its chronic reversed water-fire circulation.

One symptom of the earth's reversed water-fire energy flow is global warming, which shows that the planet's harmonious temperature balance is breaking. The earth has accumulated an incredible amount of stress from global warming, including expanding desertification, melting glaciers, rising sea levels, and abnormal climate events. The pain the earth is suffering because of human greed is boomeranging back to us. When climate change causes frequent extreme weather events—including wildfires, droughts, and flooding—wild animals lose their habitat and move into places where humans live or breed livestock. The potential for human viral infection increases as a result.

We humans have caused the planet's reversed water-fire circulation. As more and more people lose their sense of harmony and balance because of extreme stress and materialistic lives, our species' reversed water-fire flow is becoming more severe with time. Our reversed energy state is perfectly reflected in all areas of human life. First of all, personal relationships are shaken. If your chest and head are flooded with heat, that fire energy is bound to spread to others, even unknown to you, through your attitude, words, or deeds. Consequently, a vicious cycle develops in which people inflict wounds on each other, creating a reversed water-fire flow that causes people to routinely steal the energy of others and have their own energy stolen. Imagine people with reversed water-fire flow, their heads hot and bellies cold, struggling for each other's energy. We can't deny that this is an unfortunate aspect of modern human society.

This human energy state is reflected, unaltered, in people's attitude toward the global environment. They don't know how to care for their planet because their own energy is unstable. They're in pain, so they make the earth suffer, too. The results of our actions in dealing with others and the planetary environment—both of which arise out of our energy state—come back to haunt us. It is obvious that the earth's reversed water-fire energy flow will continue intensifying if humanity doesn't change its ways. Unless the water-fire flow of humanity is restored, the water-fire balance of the planet will not be maintained.

If the Planet Hurts, So Do You

Just as we should live balanced water-fire energy lifestyles—taking care of our bodies and minds, and discarding the thought that drugs, doctors, or insurance will take care of our health for us—each of us should become caretakers for the planet, ensuring that the earth has good water-fire energy flow. It won't be effective enough to wait for environmental policymakers to solve the planet's health problems. Let's remember that we humans were the ones who reversed the earth's water-fire energy flow, and we humans will have to be the ones who will correct it.

We can live without a country, religion, or ideology, but we cannot exist if our environment is sick and we're unable to breathe the air, drink the water, or eat the food it provides. When nature gets sick, human beings also get sick. If the water-fire energy balance of nature is broken, preventing water and air from circulating as they should, then human water-fire energy circulation can't be adequately maintained, either.

It's important to recover our sense for achieving harmony and balance for the sake of the planet's health. The natural environment is being ruined now because our will to control ourselves has weakened. When we lose our sense of balance, we search endlessly for novel and more potent stimuli to keep us constantly entertained and distracted from our situation. We use more energy and resources, and create more waste in the process. In our present way of life, our drive for individual satisfaction creates the earth's stress.

The natural healing ability and sense of balance within us are not human-made. They've been given to us from the beginning of our lives—like water, like air. When we recover these qualities, hidden within everyone, we will succeed both at taking care of our bodies and at looking after nature. Living in a way that allows you to sustain your water-fire energy balance is good for the entire ecosystem of the earth.

Listening to your body and awakening your physical senses is waking up your sense for communicating with nature. Why? Because our bodies are nature. We feel nature when we feel our breathing and our energy. If we feel and love nature inside us, we feel and focus more on nature outside us.

Creating a Balanced Water-Fire Energy Lifestyle

During the COVID-19 pandemic, the whole world experienced unprecedented hardships and suffering, but with them have come changes and new opportunities. While humanity paused, nature started breathing again. As industrial and social activities decreased, the sky—once ashen with atmospheric pollution—turned blue again in many urban areas. Sea turtles that had been forced off the beaches by waves of human visitors came back to lay eggs. Although a huge problem, this crisis has shown us that even environmental degradation, which used to make us feel helpless and weigh us down, offering no hint of a solution, can reverse itself if given the chance. Seeing nature purifying itself at an amazing pace when free of human interference, we realize once again how great the power of nature is in finding its own balance and stability.

Physical distancing because of the pandemic also brought closures and disruptions in many areas of our lives. This applies to relationships between communities and countries, as well as relations between individuals. Fundamentally, however, we've become keenly aware of how connected the world is—how much we want to connect and communicate, and how essential it is for the health and safety of each of us to care for other people and our communities. In the offline world, we've headed into a contactless era because of the corona pandemic. The offline world has become a bit lonely, a place without much face-to-face interaction, but the online world has become more closely and efficiently interconnected than ever, transcending the limitations of space and offering new hope for humanity.

The big problems currently threatening the sustainability of the earth and humanity—environmental pollution, nuclear threats, wealth inequality—cannot be solved by the power of any one country or group. The very nature of the problem is global, so it can be resolved only through connection and cooperation. During the pandemic, most countries chose to shut down, not allowing foreign travelers to visit, to prioritize the protection of their own citizens. So in a way, people became more isolated and separated than before. But to deal with a contagious disease threatening the entire human species, countries will have to connect and cooperate as never before. Our survival depends on it.

We must not forget the simple truth that everything is inter-connected. The wisdom of connecting and communicating through breathing, the key tool of water-fire energy circulation, teaches us this. The essence of breathing is rhythm and balance. If you've inhaled, you must exhale. If you hold one breath, not wanting to let it go, you won't be able to take in the next breath, thereby disrupting life's rhythm. Circulation continues only if you exhale as much as you've inhaled—given back as much as you've received.

This applies to our relationships with people and with nature, as well. When you give more, more comes in, and the amount of energy available grows. The unspoken agreement behind most human interactions goes something like this: "If you give to me first, then I'll give to you." Nature, however, always gives to us first, without demanding anything in return. If we learn even a little from nature, we'll be able to have a mindset that thinks of the self and the whole together, and we'll be able to create more virtuous cycles among ourselves by first giving and doing what's needed.

Feeling the rhythm of life coming and going with our breath, we can ask ourselves these questions: How much do I care for and look after my body, which is with me my entire life? What value do I add to my community? What am I contributing to the earth and nature, which provide me a base for life?

If the value we contribute is less than the value we enjoy, or if we cause harm rather than contribute, that debt will come back to haunt us. It will destroy the foundation of our lives.

The year 2020 was an extraordinary and peculiar time. On a massive scale, we have all been focused on what's happening in our communities and the world as a whole, not just ourselves. What kinds of changes will these intense and unusual experiences bring us—experiences that we've all had, and that continue even now?

We might continue the same patterns of life we had before, a life of reversed water-fire energy circulation. We might continue to repeat things that ruin our health and the health of the planet. Or we might create a new lifestyle of water-fire energy balance in which healthy circulation and win-win approaches are possible, both for our personal lives and for the earth. Whatever happens, of this I am certain: the power to create such changes is never found on the outside. It depends on what each of us does, and it starts with the changes we make within ourselves and in our daily lives. Good water-fire circulation in each of us can accelerate such change. When humanity recovers Water Up, Fire Down energy flow, the earth recovers it as well. That is our hope.

Acknowledgments

With every book I have the privilege to publish, I am always sincerely grateful to the many talented people who help make it a physical reality. This book was made possible by the brilliant editing of the Korean manuscript by Jiyoung Oh, Hyerin Moon, and Steve Kim, and its translation by Daniel Graham. Nicole Dean and Phyllis Elving gave the English manuscript its refined elegance and clarity, while Eunjung Shin added lively illustrations. Kiryl Lysenka designed the powerful cover and interior design, and Michela Mangiaracina polished the interior and gave it the finishing touches.

I'm also grateful for the various individuals who gave feedback and advice during the publishing process and for the many unnamed people who have experienced the Water Up, Fire Down energy principle and shared their stories with me.

About the Author

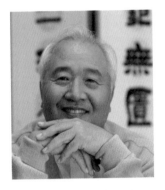

Ilchi Lee is a visionary, mentor, and educator, who has devoted his life to teaching energy principles and developing methods to nurture the full potential of the human brain.

For the last four decades, his mission has been to help people harness their creative power. For this goal, he developed mind-body training methods such as Body & Brain Yoga and Brain Education, which have inspired many people around the world to live healthier and happier lives. He also founded the undergraduate Global Cyber University and the graduate University of Brain Education.

Lee has penned more than 40 books, including the *New York Times* bestseller *The Call of Sedona: Journey of the Heart*, as well as *The Power Brain: Five Steps to Upgrading Your Brain Operating System* and *I've Decided to Live 120 Years: The Ancient Secret to Longevity, Vitality, and Life Transformation.*

A well-respected humanitarian, Ilchi Lee has been working

with the United Nations and other organizations for global peace through his nonprofit International Brain Education Association (IBREA Foundation). He began the Earth Citizen Movement, a global drive to raise awareness of the value of living mindfully and sustainably as a steward of the earth, and started the nonprofit Earth Citizens Organization (ECO). For more information about Ilchi Lee, visit Ilchi.com.

Resources

Ilchi Lee's Email Newsletter

Ilchi Lee sends weekly inspirational messages and meditations for managing your energy and your mind to master your life. Get ongoing advice for centering your mind on your true nature. Sign up at Ilchi.com/newsletter.

Body & Brain Yoga and Tai Chi Classes

For help creating and maintaining Water Up, Fire Down energy balance from experienced instructors, visit one of the 100 Body & Brain Yoga and Tai Chi centers across the United States. Group classes, workshops, and individual sessions are available both online and offline. Find a center near you at BodynBrain.com.

ChangeYourEnergy.com

This website is a leading online educational platform and lifestyle product store based on Ilchi Lee's teachings. It provides video courses, articles, and weekly live classes and webinars for all levels on energy management and meditation.

Books of Related Interest

The following books have useful information to deepen your Water Up, Fire Down energy practice. See them all and more of Ilchi Lee's books at BestLifeMedia.com.

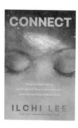

CONNECT

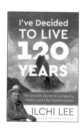

I'VE DECIDED TO LIVE 120 YEARS

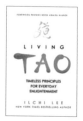

LIVING TAO

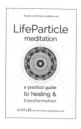

LIFEPARTICLE MEDITATION

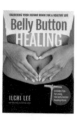

BELLY BUTTON HEALING

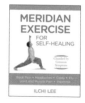

MERIDIAN EXERCISE FOR SELF-HEALING

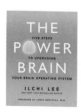

THE POWER BRAIN

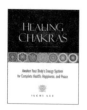

HEALING CHAKRAS

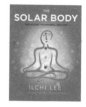

THE SOLAR BODY